ALZHEIMER'S DISEASE
Policy and practice across Europe

Edited by

Morton Warner
Sally Furnish
Marcus Longley
and
Brian Lawlor

Foreword by

Silvia
Queen of Sweden

T0138954

Radcliffe Medical Press

Radcliffe Medical Press Ltd
18 Marcham Road
Abingdon
Oxon OX14 1AA
United Kingdom

www.radcliffe-oxford.com
The Radcliffe Medical Press electronic catalogue and online ordering facility.
Direct sales to anywhere in the world.

British Library Cataloguing in Publication Data

A catalogue record for this book is available from the British Library.

ISBN 1 85775 416 6

Typeset by Aarontype Limited, Easton, Bristol
Printed and bound by TJ International Ltd, Padstow, Cornwall

Contents

Foreword

Over the past ten years increasing attention has been given to the needs of patients suffering from dementia, their families and carers. Most important of all has been the general change of attitude to a more analytical and positive approach, e.g. the demand for correct diagnosis, medication, treatment and housing. The aim is no longer cure but the prospect of living life to its fullest potential, even with the handicap of dementia.

Quality of life has many dimensions. Physical, mental, social and spiritual suffering and pain can be hard to express if you are suffering from dementia. And still we have to endeavour to understand the complex problems of all the different faces of dementia. We have to tackle the problems of the family and of the care-givers. Any illness causes anxiety. The demented patient tends to be left alone. As a family, your burden is heavy when caring for a loved, demented close relative. There are more questions than answers, more pain and grief than comfort and support.

The long period of the family's bereavement is a part of the terminal pain and mourning. Not only the family but also staff members may find themselves suffering from a feeling of helplessness and exhaustion. All the time you do your best and still you feel it is not sufficient.

Alzheimer's disease, together with all other kinds of dementia, is very common all over the world. This book, containing reports from the 15 different countries of the European Union, will be a great help for all to improve conditions for sufferers as well as carers, in Europe and elsewhere. It gives rise to three hopes in my mind.

My first hope is that all those in many fields of medicine who have in their care patients with incurable brain diseases will find this book valuable and well worth reading. Advances and initiatives in the field of treatment are important to follow up and are now likely to come not only from the traditional university hospital setting but also from special units, teams or schools teaching what dementia is – how to diagnose it, how to give optimal care or how to stimulate important research.

My next hope is that this book will make it easier to do so. Demented people are usually old, are less able to care for themselves and have more long-term problems than people suffering from most other diseases. Do we see their needs? Do we learn? Do we still remember 'to cure sometimes, to relieve often, to comfort always'? Patients are excellent teachers. They are both receiving and giving, they are both strong and weak. They are like you and me, human beings, only with more diverse needs and a new behaviour. Do we recognise the care-givers strain associated with the changed behaviour of their loved ones, their own feelings of loss and their new role in life?

My final hope is that you will give every one of these patients, and their families, of your interest, knowledge, time and love. Only then can we dare to live with confidence to our very end.

Silvia
Queen of Sweden
Drottningholm
May 2001

About the contributors

Michel Aberlen
SEDI
Paris

Christine Flori
SEDI
Paris

Sally Furnish
Head of Clinical Psychology
Mersey Care NHS Trust
Rathbone Hospital, Liverpool

Jean Georges
Executive Director
Alzheimer Europe, Luxembourg

Dianne Gove
Information Officer/Project Manager
Alzheimer Europe, Luxembourg

Margaret Kelleher
Consultant in Old Age Psychiatry
St Camillus Hospital, Limerick

Brian Lawlor
Consultant Psychiatrist
St Patrick's and St James's Hospitals, Dublin

Marcus Longley
Senior Fellow and Associate Director
Welsh Institute for Health and Social Care

David McDaid
Research Officer in LSE Health and Social Care
London School of Economics and Political Science

Leen Meulenberg
Scientific Collaborator
Belgian Inter-university Center on Health Research and Action, Brussels
Co-ordinator of the Mental Health Assessment Taskforce of WHO/EURO

Joanna Murray
Senior Lecturer in Mental Health and Ageing
Institute of Psychiatry, King's College London

Greg Swanwick
Consultant Psychiatrist in the Psychiatry of Old Age
South Western Area Health Board and Adelaide & Meath Hospital

Morton Warner
Professor of Health Policy and Strategy
University of Glamorgan
Director, Welsh Institute for Health and Social Care

Acknowledgements

The editors gratefully acknowledge the co-operation of the chapter authors in the developmental work, which was vital to the production of this book. In their turn, the authors pay tribute to their many colleagues throughout Europe who worked with them on the original research upon which the chapters are based. Particular thanks also go to Lisa Griffiths and Rosemary Scadden for their tireless efforts and good humour in processing the various drafts.

Our request to Sylvia, Queen of Sweden, to write a foreword met with an instant response from one who had personal involvement with Alzheimer's disease. We thank her for this and the continuing interest she shows.

All of the work reported and discussed here was funded by the European Commission.

1

Alzheimer's disease: an introduction to the issues

Marcus Longley and Morton Warner

What is Alzheimer's disease?

In 1907, a 51-year-old woman died in Germany after suffering from dementia. A post mortem examination was carried out, which revealed that her brain was highly abnormal when compared with non-demented women of the same age. In particular, the pathologist found it was shrunken in size, many of its cells had died and disappeared, while others contained 'dense bundles of fibrils'. Throughout the brain, there were deposits of a 'peculiar substance'. The pathologist's name was Alois Alzheimer, and this was the first diagnosed case of a disease that now is known to affect 1 in 20 people over the age of 65 in Europe, with this rate doubling every five years between the ages of 65 and 95.

Alzheimer's disease (AD) is the commonest form of dementia, accounting for between one-half and two-thirds of all cases. Its causes are still largely unknown, although a variety of factors are probably involved, including age, genetic factors, other diseases, lifestyle, environment, head injuries, and even level of education. It knows no social boundaries, as the authorship of the Foreword shows, and brings about feelings of despair and compassion from all who come into contact with sufferers.

AD leads to a progressive decline in the ability to remember, to learn, to think and to reason, and sufferers have difficulty finding and using the right words, and in recognising people, places and objects. Ewart Myer, a 78-year-old carer, described the problem as follows:

A person with Alzheimer's lives in a span of a few seconds. They cannot relish the past; they have nothing to look forward to; they live in a world of illogic.

Alice Zilonka, aged 73, had AD herself, and described her state even more succinctly:

My mind is like a dark thunderstorm.

The disease progresses at different rates in different individuals, but a broad time-line of development has been established – *see* Table 1.1. The sufferer's personality can change out of all recognition, often with a particular personality trait becoming grossly exaggerated. In its most advanced stages, the dementia results in almost total destruction of the brain's ability to function, with the sufferer becoming more and more withdrawn, and almost unable to control their behaviour.

The onset of the condition is insidious, and early symptoms are often not recognised, being mistaken for general signs of ageing. Forgetfulness is perhaps the most common cause for alarm in relatives and friends. There is no easy test to establish whether someone has AD, short of a

Table 1.1: Time-line for development of AD

	Perhaps 20 years	*3–5 years*	*3–5 years*	*5–8 years*	
	Pre-clinical stage	*Early clinical stage*	*Middle clinical stage*	*Late clinical stage*	*Death*
Symptoms		• Mild memory loss for recent events and word finding difficulties • Deterioration in higher order instrumental activities of daily living (e.g. money management)	• More obvious memory difficulties • Receptive and expressive language problems • Gradual erosion of all instrumental activities of daily living, needing supervision at home	• Continued loss of short- and long-term memory, loss of ability to communicate verbally • Problems with basic activities of daily living (dressing, toileting, feeding) • Deterioration in mobility	• Death from pneumonia or other infection

post mortem examination. The task of the doctor making the diagnosis in a living patient is made more difficult by the fact that the symptoms of early onset AD are similar to those of several other conditions – depression, vitamin deficiency and thyroid problems, for example. Diagnosis therefore usually involves a process of measuring the patient's mental state, and then of eliminating the other possible causes of the symptoms.

At present there is no cure for AD, and the symptomatic treatments are of limited benefit to most patients, especially in the middle and later stages of the disease. Help therefore tends to focus on maintaining an environment which places least stress on the sufferer, and most importantly offering whatever help is necessary for the carer. Once the diagnosis has been made, it is possible for the sufferer and their family to plan ahead and to anticipate – and therefore minimise – the future impact of the disease on all concerned. Support for carers takes a wide variety of forms, from providing information and advice, to practical help with basic caring tasks and respite from the constant burden of care.

Most carers are women, although a significant number of men are also caring for their spouses. The motivations and rewards of caring are often substantial, but so too is the burden, tinged as it often is with regret, depression, and feelings of loss as a carer's loved one changes in front of them. The following descriptions, from a 39-year-old caring for her husband with AD, and from a daughter caring for her mother, are typical of many:

> *The silence is deafening and the loneliness shattering. I remember the times when my husband and I would sit down with the crossword, gossip over an evening out with friends and discuss simple things like our children and our retirement plans. I miss those aspects of our relationship more than I can say.*

> *Mother was always the cheerful, outgoing person in the family. We knew she was becoming forgetful but the worse thing is that she doesn't want to do anything any more. She doesn't do her hair, she doesn't keep the house tidy, she absolutely won't go out.*

What makes AD different?

Every disease and disability poses challenges to the responsible professionals and policy-makers, and exacts high costs from those who suffer from it and their carers. AD, however, is different from most others, and therefore deserves special attention from policy-makers and professionals.

Table 1.2:   Top ten leading causes of DALYs given in millions in 2020 (baseline scenario, both sexes)

Rank	Disease or injury	Disability Adjusted Life Years	Cum. %
Developed regions			
	All causes	160.5	
1	Ischaemic heart disease	18.0	11.2
2	Cerebrovascular disease	9.9	17.4
3	Unipolar major disorder	9.8	23.5
4	Trachea, bronchus and lung cancers	7.3	28.0
5	Road traffic accidents	6.9	32.3
6	Alcohol use	6.1	36.1
7	Osteoarthritis	5.6	39.5
8	**Dementia, and other degenerative and hereditary CNS disorders**	**5.5**	**43.0**
9	Chronic obstructive pulmonary disease	4.9	46.0
10	Self-inflicted injuries	3.9	48.4

Source: *

Three key features of the disease are particularly relevant. First, there is the progressive nature of the condition. This makes early detection difficult, demands different levels of response from health and social care services as time goes by, and requires long-term commitment from carers. Secondly, there is no cure, and little effective treatment. This all too often encourages health and social care agencies and professionals to place too little priority on AD services, passing too much of the responsibility for care onto family members. This is compounded by paying too little attention to the needs of carers in service planning processes: two-thirds of dementia sufferers are cared for at home. Thirdly, the numbers of those with AD will increase significantly in the coming years, as the population ages.

In all, it is a major issue which will assume even greater importance in the future. Some significant work has been completed recently which quantifies the burden of disease likely to accrue in the early part of the next century.* Table 1.2 shows that AD, as one of the neuro-degenerative group, will feature highly.

Alzheimer's disease – a paradox

Across Europe there is a fundamental paradox at the heart of our attitude as a society towards AD. On the one hand, there is general

* Murray CJL and Lopez AD (eds) (1996) *Quantifying Global Health Risks: estimates of the burden of disease attributable to selective risk factors.* Harvard Press, Cambridge, MA.

recognition that people with the condition (and other dementias) receive a generally poor level of service in comparison with other groups; and yet, on the other hand, there is little sign of any determined attempt to improve the situation. Such paradoxes are far from being unique in public policy. It is upon an understanding of the reasons for the paradox that future progress depends, and part of the answer lies in the low status accorded to this group of people.

Although the member states differ considerably in terms of their policies and services for people with AD and dementia generally, it remains the case that every state accords this client group relatively low status. There are many indicators of this, such as the absence of planning processes and policies specifically targeted at the group, the relatively low prestige enjoyed by many doctors, nurses and other healthcare professionals working with demented patients, and the ambivalent nature – bordering on social stigma – typical of much popular media coverage of dementia, both factual and fictional. This low status underlies many of the other issues described in this book.

The causes of this low status are many and various. They include:

- the often ambiguous attitude of society at large to its older members – a complex mixture of respect, love and sympathy, coupled with contempt, fear and lack of understanding
- the 'invisibility' of the problem, in part a consequence of the marginalised position of most patients, effectively denied a public voice by the consequences of their condition
- the willingness – at least hitherto – of most families of people with dementia to arrange for the care of the affected relative without demanding more resources
- the lack of good models of service provision emerging from the past – partly because dementia has only relatively recently become a major public policy issue as the population has aged
- the fact that there is no cure, which tends to conflict with the overriding medical (and other health professionals') aim to save life
- the concern of Ministries of Finance and insurance companies that the burgeoning numbers of demented people, coupled with the low level of historical provision for them, might lead to an explosion of demand for services which cannot easily be afforded.

Many of the above are, of course, interrelated.

To see how the paradox is sustained in practice, consider the position relating to the early diagnosis of dementia. The intellectual and humanitarian case for early identification of people with AD is well established. And yet, many policy-making organisations, as well as individual practitioners, still do not accept this; or if they do, seem unable or unwilling to bring it about. This is partly a consequence of the generally low status of AD. But there are also more specific causes. Many professionals lack the relevant skills or time to perform the differential diagnosis necessary, or can see little point in so doing, given the limited possibility of doing what they most want to do, i.e. preserve life. There may also be an argument that the patient's best interests – in terms of preserving their dignity or confidentiality – are not best served by making an early diagnosis. Relatives, too, will often collude with professionals and request that the diagnosis not be disclosed to the patient, further underscoring family members' negative attitudes to Alzheimer's disease. In such a way, thousands of well-meaning people – professional and lay – sustain the paradox.

Inequity between member states of the EU

It is often difficult to compare the quality of healthcare provision across Europe, given the very diffcrent organisational and philosophical contexts in which the member states work. In the case of AD, however, such comparisons are made somewhat easier by the fact that there is such a high measure of agreement on the basic characteristics of good service provision and policy for AD. It is possible, therefore, to map the extent to which individual member states fall short of the ideal.

There are many examples of inequity of provision of dementia care within and across the different member states. Clinical practice models are quite advanced in some countries but are embryonic or at an early stage of development in others. Even in those where dementia care practice is well developed, there is often geographical inequity in the provision of such services, or imbalances in the level of specialist provision, that translate into inequity for the sufferers and their carers. In most member states, primary care personnel are significantly under-trained and under-resourced to deal with the rising tide of dementia sufferers, contributing to late detection and treatment.

Funding mechanisms, drug reimbursement procedures and prescribing for new drug treatments in AD vary from country to country and represent another source of inequity for patients and their carers. AD and dementia are almost unique among the leading causes of chronic disability and ill health in that the sufferers themselves are most often not able to act as advocates for the treatment of their condition. This may partly account for the low priority given in some member states to the funding of new treatments and interventions for this condition.

No state, then, has a perfect level of provision, and there is room for improvement in all. It is also true, however, that some have managed to develop better provision than others. This is often explained by such basic issues as the strength of the local economy (as a key determinant of the level of expenditure on welfare); but, whatever the cause, there is a clear *prima facie* need for co-ordination of services and policies to reduce current inequities.

'Joining up' services and policies

Alzheimer's disease patients have a multiplicity of different, and often quite intractable, problems. There is much attention paid now to the need for multidisciplinary health and social care, and for the application of both medical and social models of care, and nowhere is this more needed than in the case of services for people with AD. A whole range of professional disciplines and skills must be brought to bear at the appropriate junctures. Box 1.1 itemises these.

Such multidisciplinary working, across many agencies, requires considerable co-ordination – the various elements need to be 'joined up' into a coherent whole, focused primarily on the needs of the clients.

It is not that multi-agency dementia services do not exist, but that policies frequently do not support their development or continuation, and

---

Box 1.1: Elements of service provision

Home care service	Domestic support, domiciliary nursing, auxiliary nursing
Primary care teams	General practitioner, nurse, therapist, assessment and care planning
Social care	Social workers, assessment and care planning
Day care	Support worker in own home, social care, hospital-based (decreasing)
Respite care	In own home, unit/centre
Secondary service	Psycho-geriatrician, geriatrician, neurologist
Long-term nursing homes	For-profit, charitable
Hospitals	Psychiatric units, geriatric and general
Long-term residential homes	State (decreasing), for-profit, voluntary, religious
Voluntary sector	Domiciliary, support workers in own home

other priority groups take precedence. Good demonstration projects for dementia services have existed in a number of countries for some time, but they have not generally had much impact on policy formulation.

The best match of service to need will often be achieved by addressing the issue of appropriate specialisation. All European healthcare systems depend to some extent upon generalist professionals identifying the healthcare needs of the population, and meeting most of those needs themselves. In the case of AD, generalists must be able and willing to perform the majority of assessments, and to provide continuity of care to the patient and their carers throughout the progression of their disease. If they are to fulfil this role effectively, however, they must also have easy access to the sorts of specialist service which it is not practicable to provide at the primary care level. Deficiencies in both sectors must be addressed simultaneously. Policies directed towards co-ordinating services through a form of primary care, together with social care planning and defined pathways into secondary specialist services, are particularly important for the future direction of services.

Policy-makers, too, need to work across their own boundaries in respect of this particular group of people. In fact, *most* government departments formulate and implement policy which can improve – or make more difficult – the lives of people with AD and their carers. Such departments include social security, transport and housing, as well as the more obvious health and social services. Most member states have examples of situations where policy formulated for another group – such as those with physical disabilities – is being applied to the circumstances of those with dementia, with the inevitable results. What is needed is policy specifically formulated to meet the unique circumstances of dementia, and which embraces all relevant departments and agencies.

Again, as so often in discussions about AD, one returns to the issue of priorities: co-ordination could be achieved, if only it were accorded sufficient attention amongst policy-makers and service providers. The pre-existing boundaries, which make little sense from the perspective of AD patients and their carers, usually serve other valid administrative purposes. Therefore the objective should be either to develop mechanisms for bridging the divides in this instance, or to create entirely new arrangements for patients with dementia. The preferred option will depend upon the individual local circumstances, but the degree of priority should universally be high.

National governments would be assisted in this task if there were more effective means of disseminating throughout Europe the lessons of practice development and the models of organisation employed in different countries.

Caring for the carers

There is a considerable body of evidence to show that the carers of elderly people with dementia have poorer physical and emotional health than carers of elderly people who are equally dependent but less affected by deteriorating mental capacity. Also, a higher proportion of family caring situations break down irretrievably when the carer of an elderly person with dementia becomes unwell themselves for a period of time. Frequently, services provided on a crisis basis are less effective in maintaining the person with dementia than family care-givers, and this is even true of elderly spouse carers. It is very much in the best interests of services to support any existing carers before they cease to be able to cope.

The structure of this book

Although the emphasis of each chapter is different, two common themes recur throughout. The first is that dementia in general, and AD in particular, poses a set of challenges to policy-makers different from those of any other form of disability. The differences are numerous, as exemplified in each chapter, and together they demand a tailor-made approach to AD. The second theme is that of complexity – the needs of sufferers and their carers are enormously varied, and can only be met by a co-ordinated approach, both to policy and to implementation. While these messages are disarmingly simple, policy-makers and others still fail to appreciate their profound implications for public policy towards dementia. Chapter 2 sets out this policy context in some detail.

Dianne Gove expands on this in Chapter 3, exploring a number of the most important ethical and legal issues, and drawing on work undertaken by Alzheimer Europe, the umbrella organisation of Alzheimer's Associations across the continent. This completes the background against which the other chapters are set. In particular, she shows how the challenging nature of diagnosis of AD presents professionals with unique dilemmas relating to its disclosure, and how this is dealt with in the different member states. She goes on to discuss how various approaches to the legal framework surrounding AD have developed across Europe, with very different philosophies of responsibility for care exhibited between, for example, southern Europe and Scandinavia. She concludes with a discussion of the legal mechanisms which states have put in place to protect people with AD, from themselves and from others.

Chapter 4 explores two complementary approaches to conceptualising 'carer burden', and in the process refines the term considerably. Joanna Murray and Dave McDaid take the perspectives of the psychologist and the health economist, respectively, and discuss both the rewards and the costs of caring for someone with AD. Neither perspective proves to be sufficient in itself to capture the complexity of the bond which ties carer to sufferer, but together they offer the policy-maker a set of insights to inform the sort of 'joined-up' policy which is so urgently needed in this area.

Sally Furnish, in Chapter 5, focuses on the services currently in place to meet the health and social needs of people with AD and their carers, and on how better models of service provision are being developed in Europe. She explores how the degree of consensus on what constitutes good practice can be combined with the experience of developing model services on a small scale, to achieve the core elements of a service model fit for European application, supported by appropriate policy initiatives.

Brian Lawlor, Greg Swanwick and Margaret Kelleher in Chapter 6 report on clinical practice across Europe in both primary and secondary care, looking critically at the state of development. At best, practice is adequate, but the policy agenda in terms of training for skilled assessment, provision of specialist care and the establishment of an accessible practice research database is even more challenging.

In Chapter 7, Christine Flori and Michel Aberlen identify the training and development needs of staff currently providing mainly *social* care. They argue that the quality of life both of people with AD and of the carers themselves could be greatly enhanced by a concerted move across Europe to broaden and deepen the training provided for this often neglected workforce.

The power of information to change most aspects of health and social services is the subject of considerable speculation throughout Europe. In Chapter 8, Dave McDaid, Jean Georges and Leen Meulenberg examine the current deficits in the provision of information to professionals and lay people, and how they could be resolved. They also look over the horizon to see how these needs could be better met by the new information technologies of the coming years.

Finally, in Chapter 9, Morton Warner and Sally Furnish consider how Europe might move towards greater 'coherence' in policy and practice across the member states. This they define as being about consistency of approach and reasoning, rather than the final destination of 'convergence' of policy. The chapter concludes with a statement of 12 new coherencies which require urgent attention.

2

The national policy context across Europe

Marcus Longley and Morton Warner

Introduction

The growth in the prevalence of dementia over the last few years has been constant and steady, linked with demographic changes in the European population that show a rise in the number of elderly people. In Britain alone, estimates suggest that there are between 0.5 and 1 million people suffering from some form of dementia. There is also evidence to suggest that Alzheimer's disease (AD) is the most common form of dementia and accounts for 50% of all classified cases. It is thought that 6.2% of the 1996 UK population aged 65+ will have some form of cognitive disability. Of these, 36% are estimated to be resident in institutional care, where they make up half of the residents. Data generated by the Eurodem Study reveal similar prevalence estimates for the rest of Europe.[1] It is also clear from these figures that the prevalence of both dementia and cognitive impairment increases dramatically with age.

The uniqueness of the problems of caring for an older person with cognitive impairment means that in both formal and informal care situations specialist skills and facilities are required, even for apparently simple problems. The complexity of the different needs of people suffering from dementia makes the question of provision of services problematic. Hence the European Parliament's decision to provide new funding specifically for the study of Alzheimer's and other neuro-degenerative diseases in Europe in 1996.

Recent history of policy developments

The most striking feature to emerge from a review of the recent history of policy in this area is the movement towards a substantial degree of agreement on key principles of policy. Many of these are now enshrined in the policy frameworks of all member states, and others have been adopted in most countries.

This convergence has taken place only within the last 10–15 years, with different countries moving at different rates towards the current position of near consensus. The driving forces fall into two categories:

Politico-economic

Policy has been driven by a recognition of the rapidly growing demands of older people in general (largely as a result of their increasing numbers), and of older people with dementia in particular, and the financial and political implications of failing to provide the most cost-effective patterns of state and other support for them and their carers. For example, all member states share similar future demographic profiles (increasing numbers of elderly – and very elderly – people, and a decline in the proportion of people of working age); this, combined with research evidence of the prevalence of dementia, quickly revealed a potential future problem. In some states, such as Finland, one particular epidemiological study, the Mini-Finland Study,[2] published in 1985, marked the beginning of a substantial re-evaluation of the scale of future needs; in others, a series of official reports contributed to the change.

Humanitarian

There has emerged a general recognition that the *quality* of support provided in the past is no longer acceptable. Key developments here have been both professionally-led (for example, Health Advisory Service reports in the UK) and led by bodies more central to national political structures – for example, the 1988 National Health Council Report in the Netherlands.[3] Closely linked with these has been the growth of patients' and carers' representative groups, notably the Alzheimer's disease societies, and a growing articulation of the values and priorities of older people in general.

In many respects, developments in policy towards Alzheimer's patients and families reflect the development of broader health and social welfare policies for older people – the same policy drivers operate across all patient groups. However, different emphases and different conclusions have emerged to meet the particular circumstances of this group of people. Also, in many countries two somewhat separate policy 'streams' have converged to produce current policy: the framework developed for people with mental illness (with a particular emphasis on protection for those who are unable to safeguard their own affairs), and policies towards older people (with an emphasis on maintaining independence).

The principles which have emerged to underlie public policy can therefore be summarised as shown in Table 2.1.

Table 2.1: Key principles that have emerged to inform national policy frameworks

Principles emphasised by all member states	*Principles emphasised by most member states*
1 People with dementia should be enabled to remain at home for as long as possible	1 There should be a systematic attempt to equate service provision with need
2 Carers should receive as much help as possible, in order to facilitate 1 above	2 Categorical care should be replaced by care which addresses the general needs of sufferers
3 Sufferers should retain maximum control over the support they receive	3 Early diagnosis of dementia should be encouraged
4 *All* relevant services should be co-ordinated at the local level	4 The needs of people with dementia are addressed only as part of the approach to older people in general at the national level
5 Sufferers in institutional care should live in surroundings which are as 'homely' as possible	

The rate of progress towards this consensus has varied between states. Some identified the needs of older and demented people relatively early, and others much later. Amongst the first to do so was France, which in 1962 emphasised the importance of 'extended domiciliary stay', and the Netherlands, which has encouraged the development of domiciliary care since 1963. Other countries only started slowly to develop policy in the late 1960s and 1970s. During the course of the 1980s, however, the drivers identified above became much more pronounced, and policy development became much more rapid – witness the further development of policy in countries where progress had already been made, and initial stirrings in others, e.g. Catalonia, Spain from 1986, and Luxembourg, culminating in the governmental declaration of 1989.[4] The result was that by the late 1980s, most countries were espousing the principles outlined above. However, in services for dementia, as in many other aspects of health and social care provision, the rate of development has been conditioned by the total amount of resources available for such services, with the result that in countries such as Greece and Portugal, both policy and service provision for this client group has developed slowly and rather later than in other member states.

The 1990s has been a period of consolidation, during which criticism has focused not only on the policy framework, but on the perceived inadequacies of its implementation. The fact of consensus on objectives does not, of course, imply that services and other policies actually ensure the desired standard of support in each member state. A number of criticisms of the implementation, or lack of implementation, of national policy have also emerged in most member states. These have highlighted areas where the espoused principles have not resulted in desired change because of:

- continuing lack of adequate resources, particularly resources 'earmarked' specifically for this client group
- the persistent, relatively low status of dementia services in the broader context of healthcare
- inadequate attempts to ensure patient and carer control of services, which remain largely shaped by organisational and professional imperatives
- the health and social needs of patients and carers still do not always receive equal attention.

The legislative framework

None of the member states has enacted legislation relating to the specific needs and circumstances of people with dementia. Such people (and their carers) are therefore governed by legislation that attempts to address more generic situations.

Legislation falls into two main categories: that relating to the individual rights of people with dementia (much of which is written in the context of general mental illness); and that relating to the overall control of health and other services.

Individual rights

Legislation on individual rights shares several common assumptions across Europe, while of course reflecting the idiosyncrasies of different national legal systems. Such legislation is commonly relevant to the circumstances of individuals with dementia in the following cases:

- *where matters of property require resolution* – some states (e.g. the Netherlands, UK, Ireland) have specific provision for enduring powers of attorney, or 'living wills', which allow people to determine in advance how their property should be administered, and by whom, before they cease to be able to control it themselves; other states (e.g. Finland, France) do not have this provision, and seek to establish means of administering the property of demented people in a way which might best have met their wishes, once the dementia is established
- *when giving consent to treatment* – most states apply general mental health (and other) legislation where necessary to compel demented patients to receive treatment (under appropriate safeguards). Until that point is reached, however, many states enshrine in legislation the patient's right to choose between different forms of treatment. In Finland, for example, mental health legislation is also available, but until patients qualify under that law, they have a statutory right to care in accordance with their will, and if they refuse treatment or a particular procedure, they must be offered treatment in some other medically acceptable way. In France, individual rights are protected, including the patient's right to refuse hospitalisation. In some states (e.g. Luxembourg), however, specific legal guarantees of individual autonomy for dementing people are absent.
- *when seeking access to medical and other records* – many states have moved to provide certain rights of access to one's own (and a demented relative's) medical and other information: in Denmark, doctors are obliged to disclose a diagnosis of dementia to the patient.

Some states (e.g. Finland, UK) have also made statutory provision for patients' complaints procedures.

Provision of services

Legislation governing the provision of services takes three broad forms:

- *permissive* – agencies are empowered to act to meet certain needs, but the manner and extent to which they do so is left to their discretion
- *prescriptive* – certain types of provision are required
- *regulatory* – where certain types of service are provided, and the standards of that service are regulated by the law.

Most countries have a mixture of all three. In the UK, for example, health and social services authorities are often permitted to provide various general services, but are not *required* by the law to provide any more than a very loosely defined framework of care. However, this general obligation is supplemented by specific requirements under various Acts, for example to assess the circumstances of any carer providing substantial care on a regular basis, at that carer's request.[5] There is also legislation which prescribes levels of welfare payment under varying circumstances. And then there is legislation to ensure that nursing and residential homes comply with an established system of regulation.

The extent to which the last category – regulation of service provision – has developed varies considerably between countries. Some of the most developed regulatory frameworks are found in the Netherlands, where high standards of institutional residential care are enforced by law. The degree of legal prescription also varies considerably, from the rather loose situation in the UK and elsewhere, to the position, for example in Denmark, where state authorities are required by law to provide many specific services (e.g. home help, home nursing and home nursing aids).[6]

Some states (e.g. the UK) have more recently developed a legislative framework to ensure that the needs of carers are assessed (and, hopefully, met), and pressure groups in some other countries (e.g. Ireland) are pressing for similar provision.

The financial arrangements for continuing care

'Continuing care' is defined here as being all forms of continuing personal or nursing care and associated domestic services for people who are unable to look after themselves without some degree of support, whether provided in their own homes, at a day centre, or in a residential or healthcare setting.

No country makes specific provision for the continuing care needs of Alzheimer's sufferers. This can sometimes present problems, particularly when people have to qualify for support against general criteria – for example 'being in need of permanent assistance and the care of another'. Those with early dementia can appear quite independent, but still need care.

In each of the member states, a substantial proportion of the cost of continuing care is met by individuals themselves and their families. Each country has a different set of provisions for continuing care, all characterised by multiple sources of funding, and various eligibility criteria. The key dimensions, together with the range of different types of provision across Europe, are identified in Table 2.2.

Table 2.2: Key dimensions of continuing care and the types of provision experienced across Europe

Responsibility	Basis of provision	Needs addressed	Eligibility criteria	Form of support

• Individual sufferer
  – personal insurance
  – co-payment
  – full payment
• Family
  – part payment
  – full payment
• Insurance
• Local government
• National government
• Charity/ voluntary organisations
	• Legal requirement
	• Discretionary
		• Specific (e.g. housing)
		• General (e.g. income support)
			• Means tested
			• Universal
				• Cash
				• Services

This complexity of each country's system frequently presents two problems. First, it can be difficult for individuals and families to understand (and therefore claim) their full entitlements. Second, disparities in entitlement between different local authorities and insurance arrangements, added to variations in uptake, can result in inequities in funding within member states.

In most countries, the share of total expenditure borne by the state is under review. A common concern of policy in this area is to limit the future liabilities of the taxpayer for the care of the elderly in general. This is being done by exploring various mechanisms of restricting entitlement to state-financed services (by imposing stricter needs assessment criteria, or raising thresholds under means testing), or increasing the element of individual co-payment.

To what extent are finances specifically targeted to this group?

None of the member states targets significant resources specifically at services for AD. The vast majority of provision is through generic services,

either at the primary care/community level, or through more specialised services for the elderly or elderly mentally ill. As a result, precise
estimates of the total quantum available for people with AD are generally not available, although research studies in several countries have
revealed the approximate balance of resources between categories of service provision. For example, Table 2.3 shows estimates from Denmark
relating the number of people in different types of care with the total
socio-economic costs for each category.[7]

Table 2.3:   Estimated socio-economic costs of care for demented persons, Denmark, 1992

Location of care	% of total demented persons	Estimated total socio-economic cost, 1992 (DKK bn)	% total socio-economic cost of demented persons
Own home	49%	1.8	23%
General nursing homes	39%	3.6	46%
Specialised institutions for the elderly	6%	0.7	9%
Psychiatric hospitals	3%	0.6	8%
General hospitals	3%	1.1	14%

What attempts are being made to address issues of equity?

For the purposes of this chapter, 'equity' is defined in terms of a mis-
match between service provision and objectively assessed need for those
services. The main dimensions of equity so defined are:

- *access* to services – were the appropriate services available where
  they were most needed?
- *utilisation* of services – were those in greatest need actually receiving
  their appropriate share of the services available?
- *quality* of services – was the quality of available services matched to
  the needs of the people using them?

In each of the member states, policy-makers recognise the legitimacy of
equity as a guiding principle, but it is accorded varying levels of priority.
In some, such as Finland and Ireland, government policy explicitly states
the importance of ensuring that use of services is determined by need
and not ability to pay, or geographical location. In others, such as the UK

(at the time of writing) and France, the general requirement of universal provision was endorsed, although proactive attempts to reduce existing inequities were somewhat limited. In some member states, inequity is an inherent feature of the basic social support systems – in Greece, for example, people receive benefits from one of a large number of different social insurance funds, and the pension levels vary from under Euro 80 per month to more than Euro 800.

Across Europe, several common factors leading to inequity are identified by most governments. Geographical inequities tend to reflect four broad causes: basic differences in wealth and income between regions; historical patterns of unequal investment; the particular problems of providing adequate services in rural areas, where distance can be a powerful disincentive to service utilisation; and different policies and practices between local governmental and other agencies. At a fundamental level, several member states are seeking to address basic socio-economic inequality, with a focus on macro-economic policy issues, as well as pensions provision and welfare support, both for individual sufferers and their carers. Many states are attempting to redress past patterns of unequal investment through targeted investment in service development in deprived areas. Countries with substantial rural populations generally seek to make special provision, in the form of some additional finance, to meet their needs, but usually not enough to satisfy the groups representing those people.

As far as differences in local policy and practice are concerned, many central governments deploy a combination of exhortation to standardise, with increased central 'guidance' and regulation. Local authorities in some countries are themselves also seeking to improve standardisation between their various areas. In Denmark, for instance, the National Association of Local Authorities has recognised the problems which the lack of common definitions of need and service provision pose for inter-agency co-operation.[8] As a result, they have taken the initiative to establish a 'common concept and common language' for the needs of the elderly in their localities, and the services provided for them. This should enable each authority to identify and analyse the needs of their clients, describe their efforts to meet those needs, make comparisons between themselves, and improve co-ordination of care with the health sector.

Most countries exhibit 'ageism' as one cause of inequity. Like most forms of discrimination, its impact is somewhat insidious, operating both at policy-making/implementation levels and at the point of interaction between service and client, and affecting all three dimensions of equity – access, utilisation and quality. For example, there is some evidence to suggest that comparable needs in the elderly population sometimes receive less attention and resources than in younger age groups.

Specific differences between the care provided for young and old victims of coronary artery disease has been described in the UK, and some countries also report that a diagnosis of AD in the 'old elderly' often leads to less attention from service providers than the same diagnosis in the 'young elderly'. In many countries, people diagnosed with dementia below the state retirement age are also entitled to greater social benefits than those diagnosed later – a larger disability pension, for example, which is denied to those in receipt of a retirement pension.

In those countries where there is a discernible shift in the balance of care from taxation-funding to individual responsibility, there are instances of resulting increases in inequity. In Finland, for example, there is some concern that the pressure to contain state expenditure on medicines could result in the poor being denied access in the future to medicines which might slow the progress of AD. In other countries, the policy drive to reduce state-provided hospital beds for the elderly could impact on those unable to obtain full support for private institutional care.

While most countries tend to focus on the 'access' dimension of inequity, others also seek to address inequity of 'utilisation'. Clearly there is a close link between the two, but in some circumstances the mere provision of services does not ensure that they are actually used by those in greatest need of them. This has led some states to make special provision for identifying and meeting the needs of the elderly and, if necessary, taking services to them. One example of this is the requirement in some states for the needs of all older people to be re-assessed on a regular basis. Another is the case of elderly immigrant populations, where language and cultural barriers can make existing service provision difficult to access, thereby compounding the high risks of social isolation inherent in such groups. Denmark, for example, is attempting to solve this problem by increasing the number of bi-cultural social and health care staff, and making all staff aware of the particular circumstances and needs of refugees and immigrants.[9]

How are WHO Health For All (HFA) policies being applied to Alzheimer's and neuro-degenerative diseases?

Of the six broad themes within HFA, two (equity and multi-sectoral co-operation) are considered elsewhere, and one (health issues requiring international co-operation, such as pollution) is not relevant to AD. None of the remaining themes features prominently – or in most cases, at all – in member states' policies towards AD, and there is little evidence that national policies have been greatly influenced by HFA.

However, the WHO emphasis on health promotion, public involvement and primary care finds its echo in national healthcare policies and – inasmuch as they exist at all – in policies specifically addressing AD. Thus, many countries make explicit provision for health promotion for the elderly (although critics would claim insufficient provision, given the potential for *lifelong* health promotion to improve the level of health of the elderly), and all are increasingly open to the advice of the burgeoning patients' and carers' groups.

The official emphasis on primary care is evident in each country, although reflecting the difference in the organisation and structure of different healthcare systems. As far as AD is concerned, the reduction of long-stay hospital care for demented people has *de facto* increased the role of primary care, and most new service developments for this client group – regardless of their source of funding – are located in the community.

What targets have been set to achieve health and social gain for elderly people with neuro-degenerative conditions?

Two types of 'target' are evident in health and social policy development in the member states: specific policy aims related to the development of new or improved services (referred to here as *service targets*), and published intentions to achieve specified levels of health/social improvement (*health and social gain targets*). The majority of member states have not yet developed service targets which are relevant to the needs of elderly people with neuro-degenerative (ND) conditions, and none have developed a comprehensive set of health and social gain targets which adequately address the needs of elderly people in this situation. Health and social gain targets are notoriously difficult to develop for conditions where 'cure' is not usually a realistic objective. The two areas most commonly addressed in this regard – where services can realistically expect to make an impact – are personal care and the maintenance of human dignity. However, many observers argue that there is a dearth of reliable evidence relating to the effectiveness of many of the approaches and methods routinely adopted, and very little use made of systematic attempts to measure the impact on carers' quality of life.

In addition to these generic problems associated with this client group, there are three common weaknesses associated with those targets which do exist. First, most states do not distinguish between the needs of elderly people generally and the specific needs of those with ND conditions: several states have developed targets for the elderly population, but the specific requirements of ND patients are not separately identified as objectives of public policy. There are some exceptions, however. Ireland, for example, has a goal to reduce the prevalence and severity of mental illness in older people and to raise the awareness of mental health issues.[10] The action plans specific to dementia under this goal include continuing improvement in the treatment and control of hypertension in older people to reduce the risk of dementia associated with stroke, ensuring improved social and personal environments for people with dementia, and ensuring the burden of those who care at home for people with dementia is recognised and that their needs – for example in relation to support, training and respite and day care – are met.

Second, the targets are rarely quantified in a manner which would allow assessment of the extent to which they have been achieved. Two dimensions would be important here: a precise statement of the *amount* of change or improvement required, and a specific *time period* in which it is to be achieved. The UK has attempted to address this with a series of targets which specify the change required by a particular date.[11] However, this approach has also been criticised, since the precise derivation of the numerical targets is often not clear, and it is often difficult to distinguish between changes which result from the implementation of policy and those which would have occurred anyway.

Third, the decentralised and fragmented nature of health and social care provision in many states makes the achievement of national targets very difficult. Several states have attempted to alleviate this problem by seeking agreement amongst the various regional and local responsible bodies, but with mixed success. In Denmark, for example, local authorities are responsible for setting their own targets, and a recent investigation by the Ministry of Social Affairs concluded that management and collaborators' motivation is impeded by a lack of operational targets and an *ad hoc* follow-up often related to individual cases.[12] The lack of targets means that there is no satisfactory basis for feedback. This is despite the fact that four years earlier the National Association of Local Authorities in Denmark promulgated some overall goals which could be applied to all older citizens in the country.

Interrelationships with other aspects of social policy

In each of the member states, several ministries are involved in the provision of the different types of support for AD sufferers and their carers, and the situation is further complicated by the fact that both national and local/regional levels of government are involved. This results in every case in some degree of complexity of provision and therefore confusion for many of the people who are the intended beneficiaries of state assistance.

In practice, in most countries social workers or their equivalent play a crucial role for individual sufferers and their carers in identifying their potential entitlements and advising on appropriate ways of accessing them. There are also examples of successful attempts to co-ordinate the work of different national and regional government agencies with a responsibility in this area. For example, in Catalonia, the Department of Social Welfare and the Department of Health and Social Security work together to offer an integrated *Quality of Life for the Aged Programme.*

The role of national patients' and carers' organisations in informing national policy

The growing influence of Alzheimer's organisations within the member states has paralleled the development of policy in this area. To some extent this reveals a cause and effect relationship – the growth of an advocacy movement has stimulated public policy – but also, more generally, it reflects the growing strength of consumerism and of all patients'/ carers' groups. In every state there is now at least one well-established national voice for Alzheimer's carers and patients. In countries with a longer tradition of co-operation and collaboration between government and other key stakeholders/service users – such as the Netherlands and the Scandinavian countries – the user groups are proportionately stronger and more influential; in other states – such as Greece and Portugal – the Alzheimer's societies are of much more recent origin, and have still to exert great influence at the policy formulation stage.

All of the organisations have developed – or are in the process of developing – roles in the following areas:

- *service provision* – including caring services, and individual advice and advocacy facilities to ensure that carers and patients receive the services to which they are entitled
- *policy development* – drawing in part on their experience as service providers, and also on the views of their members, organisations are to varying degrees consulted by governments, and seek to influence governments by overt lobbying
- *research* – focusing on the needs of patients and carers, often with government funding.

Some concern has been voiced intermittently about the willingness of these organisations to champion the needs of sufferers when such needs occasionally come into conflict with those of carers. There has also been some concern that these organisations, dominated as they inevitably are by carers rather than sufferers, might occasionally advocate the needs of the carer more vigorously than those of the sufferer.

Conclusion

Although there is considerable variation across the EU in relation to member states' policies towards older people generally, there is a discernible general lack of priority given to the needs of those with neuro-degenerative diseases. This is despite the fact that there is widespread consensus about the characteristics of good policy and practice. It remains to be seen whether the drivers of change identified in this chapter will together force improvement in this area of policy over the coming years.

References

1 Hofman A, Rocca WA, Brayne C *et al.* (1991) The prevalence of dementia in Europe: a collaborative study of 1980–1990 findings. *Int J Epidem.* **20**: 736–48.

2 Sulkave R, Wikström J, Aromaa A *et al.* (1985) Prevalence of severe dementia in Finland. *Neurology.* **35**: 1025–9.

3 Health Council (1988) *Advice Psycho-geriatrical Clinical Pictures No. 1988.07.* Health Council, The Hague.

4 Government of Luxembourg (1989) *National Programme in Favour of Older People.* Government of Luxembourg, Luxembourg.

5   Carers (Recognition and Services) Act 1995.

6   Ministry of Social Affairs (1992) *Pensions in Denmark: main features of Danish old age policy and care for the old*. Ministry of Social Affairs, Copenhagen.

7   Felbo O, Lindahl J, Svarre-Christensen M *et al.* (1993) *Denentes vilkår: Hvad bør der gøres? En rapport om problemer, politiske målsætninger og initiativer på demensområdet*. Ældrepolitisk afdeling, Ældre Sagen, Copenhagen.

8   Lützhøft R (1996) *Ældreområdet Forslag til fælles sprog vedrørende behov og ydelser*. Kommunernes Landsforening, Copenhagen.

9   Dansk Flytningehjælp *et al.* (1996) *Omældre*. Forlaget Kommuneinformation, Copenhagen.

10 National Council on Ageing and Older People (1998) *Health Ageing Strategy*. Department of Health, Dublin.

11 Department of Health (1992) *The Health of the Nation: a strategy for England*. HMSO, London.

12 Socialministeriet (1996) *Styring af fremtiidens hjemmepleje*. Socialministeriet, Copenhagen.

3

Ethical and legal approaches to Alzheimer's disease in the EU

Dianne Gove

Introduction

It is important to consider the ethical positions which various countries across Europe take towards Alzheimer's disease (AD), and the resulting legal frameworks. This will provide a backdrop against which most subsequent activities illustrated in this report occur.

Specifically, then, this chapter examines some of the ethical and legal issues which arise when a person is diagnosed as having AD or a related disorder. These issues can be divided broadly into two. The first section deals with issues surrounding the actual diagnosis and the consequences for the person with dementia and their carers; and it starts with the question of whether the sufferer will be informed of the diagnosis. Of course, not all people with dementia are diagnosed as such, and this is of particular importance in the light of recent advances in helpful medication. Entitlement to care is also important in the decision-making process and in determining the consequences of the disease for the family.

The second section looks largely at issues related to the protection of the person with dementia against abuse; preventing the person from coming to harm (or endangering the lives of other people) whilst driving; the consequences if the individual is in full-time employment; and, finally, the issue of genetic testing, with the possibility of discrimination by insurance companies.

In most cases, legislation reflects the ethical issues involved. However, despite the different approaches in Europe, it becomes clear that legal provisions relating to the rights of people with dementia are often lagging somewhat behind public attitudes, which have changed substantially over time.

Disclosure of the diagnosis of AD

Informing the sufferer: attitudes and practice

In the course of the last decade, awareness of dementia, particularly AD, has increased considerably. Diagnostic procedures have been developed which have resulted in the possibility of detecting the disease at a much earlier stage. This, combined with recent advances in symptomatic treatments, results in individuals being more likely to be diagnosed as having AD or another form of dementia at a time when they are still able to benefit – in the early to mid-stage of the disease. Early diagnosis will enable them to make informed decisions about their future treatment and care, and sort out their financial affairs. None of this can happen if the diagnosis has not been revealed.

Although attitudes are changing, the practice of routinely informing the person with dementia varies considerably. In Scotland, for example, a survey revealed that 56% of doctors reported that, in general, they told the patient the diagnosis compared with 19% of Italian doctors.[1] In the United States, by contrast, 95% of doctors were reported by Tiraboschi et al.[2] as having stated that they would inform a hypothetical person with dementia of his/her diagnosis. There has nevertheless been an increase in the disclosure of the diagnosis which, as pointed out by Heal and Husband,[3] bears similarities with disclosure in case of cancers. In the 1960s, 90% of doctors failed to inform patients of the diagnosis of cancer, whereas by 1979 one study revealed that 97% of doctors indicated a preference for disclosure whenever possible.[4]

Heal and Husband, reporting on the situation in East Anglia, UK, also revealed that a doctor's decision to disclose the diagnosis was affected by the age of the sufferer.[3] In their study, the mean age of those who were informed was 63.2 years, compared with 71.2 years for those who were not informed; and doctors were more prone to disclose the diagnosis to sufferers with younger carers.

Whilst this could reflect an ageist attitude, there may be other reasons too. For example, despite recent developments some doctors are reluctant to give distressing information to a patient when they cannot be absolutely certain of its accuracy, particularly in the earliest stages of the disease. The distress caused by an incorrect diagnosis was recently reported on behalf of one Swiss lady who was diagnosed as having AD, only later to find out that this was incorrect. She explained that such mistakes could ruin a person's life and lead to a reduction in confidence amongst members of the medical profession. In most cases of incorrect diagnosis, the patient is found to have been suffering from depressive pseudo-dementia.[5,6] Given that depression is fairly common in people suffering from dementia, this tends to reinforce doctors' fears of the consequences of informing potential sufferers.

Disclosure to carers is also difficult. It could be considered to be in their best interests if their family is informed, as they may need advice and assistance in order to ensure appropriate care. But disclosure could also lead to conflicts of interest, both financial and personal. Informing the family without authorisation could be construed as a violation of the patient's right to a confidential relationship with their doctor.

Some studies suggest that most people have a preference for being informed. Erde *et al.*, who interviewed patients in doctors' waiting rooms found that over 90% had a preference for knowing their diagnosis.[7] In Ireland, Maguire *et al.* revealed that while 83% of relatives of people with dementia felt that the person should not be informed, 71% felt that they themselves would like to be informed should the situation ever arise.[8] In the work carried out by Heal and Husband, carers' reasons for withholding disclosure were mainly based on the fear that it would lead to distress or that the sufferer was too cognitively impaired to understand.[3] The majority of those who had decided to disclose the diagnosis had done so because the sufferer had asked to know, or needed a meaningful explanation of the problems they were encountering.

Legal provisions

There are at least four issues covered by the existing legislation on the disclosure of diagnosis in member states:

- the right to be informed of one's diagnosis
- the right to decline such information
- the obligation on doctors to explain the diagnosis in a way that the person can understand
- the right for doctors to withhold the diagnosis subject to certain conditions.

More general legal provisions of relevance to the issue of disclosure fall into two categories: access to medical files; and the right to be informed of one's state of health.

Under the Access to Health Records Act of 1990 (which applies to Scotland, England and Wales), for example, doctors are legally obliged to let patients see their medical records if they so desire. They can, however, withhold part or all of the records if the patient is not thought to be capable of understanding the application to see them, or if it seems likely that access to them would cause serious harm to their mental health. Disclosure of the diagnosis is therefore dependent on the patient taking the initiative to request access and on the doctor's judgement of the effect that such knowledge might have.

The Patient's Charter, in Scotland, on the other hand, stipulates that a person has a right to an accurate, relevant and understandable explanation of their state of health (including diagnosis, implications and treatment).[9] Similarly, the French Charter of the Hospitalised Patient states that there should be equal access to information, even in cases where the patient experiences difficulty communicating or understanding.[10] This puts the onus on the medical professional to adapt the information to the understanding of the patient; but the charter is only applicable in the hospital setting. Article 35 of the French Code of Medical Ethics allows the doctor to withhold information 'for legitimate reasons.'

With regard to disclosure of the diagnosis to the relatives of the person with dementia, the National Health Service in Scotland Code of Practice and Confidentiality of Personal Health Information does not allow disclosure without consent except in exceptional circumstances. In recognition of the particular characteristics of dementia, the Code states that the decision to disclose or withhold information about the diagnosis should be based on the best interests of the patient. Furthermore, in all cases of disclosure of a diagnosis of dementia to relatives without the consent of the patient, the Mental Welfare Commission must be informed.

The 1998 Danish Law on Patients' Legal Status is interesting in that it also contains a general clause allowing the patient to refuse information on the condition of their health and on treatment possibilities, including the risk of complications and side effects. The 1992 Finnish Act on the Status and Rights of Patients also includes a clause to prevent information being given to the patient against their will.

Legislation varies considerably throughout Europe with regard to the disclosure of the diagnosis of dementia to the sufferer or their relatives. Where legal provisions exist, they may be open to different interpretations or, in the case of codes of practice or charters, may not be legally binding.

Alzheimer Europe recently drew up a Strategy for the 3rd Millennium, the first draft of which was approved by all member associations at the 1998 annual general meeting. In this report, the need to provide people with AD with a timely and accurate diagnosis, as well as information and understanding, was stressed. It was also decided that the special role of carers and their importance in the provision of care should be recognised. This reflects the aims of the organisation and its members, which are to support both carers and patients. For this to be possible, it is necessary that both the patient and the carer be informed of the diagnosis. In order to achieve this, whilst at the same time respecting the right of people with dementia to refuse the right to know, it is essential to convince members of the medical profession of the benefits of informing the patient and his/her carers and perhaps to campaign for specific legislation on the issue of disclosure in countries where it is lacking or in some way inadequate.

Guardianship

Early detection and diagnosis may help to prevent the person with dementia from experiencing financial and administrative difficulties as a result of symptoms such as confusion, poor concentration, memory problems and difficulties with abstract thought. If the person is aware of the diagnosis, he or she can start to make provisions for the future, when the disease is at a more advanced stage and it is no longer possible to manage alone. All EU countries have some kind of system of guardianship which provides for one or more people to take care of the financial and/or personal interests of another who is no longer capable of doing so him/herself. Even within each country, there are often different possibilities, e.g. a tutor, guardian or curator.

The role and responsibilities of this person may differ according to the system chosen. In some cases, his/her power may be limited to certain transactions and permission may be needed for others. Furthermore, the type of guardianship adopted can affect the legal status of the person with dementia. The following provides a very brief overview of several systems.

Different systems of guardianship in Europe

In England, a guardian can be appointed under the 1983 Mental Health Act. This can be the nearest relative or a social worker. The guardian has the power to require the person to live in a specific place, to ensure that doctors and social workers have access to the person and to require the person to attend a particular place in order to obtain treatment. The guardian cannot, however, force the protected person to have treatment or consent to it on his/her behalf. A guardian cannot deal with the person's money or property. For this, an appointee would be needed for small amounts of money or a receiver appointed by the Court of Protection for larger sums.

In France, the different systems of guardianship affect the status of the protected person with regard to legal capacity. A *sauvegarde de justice* does not result in the loss of legal capacity, but if the protected person makes a decision which seems to be detrimental to him/herself, it would be annulled. A *tutelle*, on the other hand, results in the total loss of legal capacity, whereas a *gérant de tutelle* can act in the interests of the person, except in certain circumstances which necessitate the authorisation of the family council. According to Article 501 of the Civil Code,[11] the judge can determine that the incapacitated person retains part of his/her legal capacity for certain decisions.

In Spain, people with dementia are seldom declared incompetent, unless the person with dementia possesses a large estate, and families are reluctant to make an official statement and become involved in large amounts of paperwork. However, they may act in the interests of a person with dementia who has not been officially declared incapacitated. This is known as *de facto* custodianship. A general guardian, on the other hand, can be appointed for a person who has been declared incompetent.[12] This guardian must support the person with dementia, promote the restoration of their capacity (not applicable in the case of dementia), encourage their reintegration into society and notify the courts of their actual condition. General guardians can also manage the property of the person with dementia but need to obtain judicial permission to sell goods, abandon rights or accept inheritances. When it is decided that the person is incapacitated, the judge may appoint a curator to assist the person with certain tasks. Finally, there is also the possibility of appointing a court-appointed defender who may intervene in cases where there is a conflict of interests during the incapacitation process, and in cases where a guardian or curator cannot perform their duties. These various guardianship measures are covered by Article 215 to Article 306 of the Civil Code.

The Enduring Power of Attorney is a useful system operative in the United Kingdom and in Ireland, which enables a specified carer to carry out financial and administrative transactions on behalf of a person with dementia. Unlike the normal power of attorney, which becomes invalid once the person becomes mentally incapable, an Enduring Power of

Attorney remains valid even when the person is diagnosed as having dementia. An Enduring Power of Attorney can even be made after dementia has been diagnosed, provided that the person is deemed to be fully aware of what is involved.

The German system of guardianship is particularly flexible and not unnecessarily restrictive. It is based on the *Betreuungsgesetz* of 1992, and has replaced previous legislation on guardianship.[13] The present law places emphasis on care and personal welfare, rather than the withdrawal of legal rights. It is very flexible, in that a judge determines which areas will be covered by the guardianship and also the extent to which the protected person retains his or her legal capacity. The guardian (*Betreuer*) can make decisions on behalf of the protected person, but an authorisation from the judge is required for certain decisions, e.g. high risk medical decisions, decisions concerning internment, deprivation of liberty or the sale of property. The same guardian can, nevertheless, deal with financial and non-financial decisions. Alternatively, several guardians can be appointed. An important feature of the *Betreuungsgesetz* is that provisions are made to support guardians in their task. A guardian can seek advice from the guardianship court for all questions relating to civil law and from the relevant authorities for questions relating to assistance, e.g. social services, meals on wheels, the availability of residential care etc. Authorities are in fact responsible for the provision of adequate initiation and training courses for guardians.

A similar system has been recently implemented in Denmark.[14] Previous legislation consisted of an either/or approach to incapacity, whereas the new law, like the German system, gears the guardianship to the needs and particular situation of the person with dementia. Guardianship can be limited to economic conditions or personal relations, according to the requirements of the person with dementia. As with the German system, the guardianship should not be more extensive than is actually necessary.

Supervision and control with regard to guardianship

One problem with guardianship in many countries is that there is very little if any control of the guardian once appointed. Consequently, it is possible for a guardian to abuse their position, particularly in cases where they are handling a person's financial affairs. Economic exploitation and theft is one form of abuse to which old people are particularly prone.[15] This is a potential problem with the Enduring Power of Attorney in England, Wales, Scotland and Ireland. Despite its usefulness, it cannot be revoked by the donor once he or she has become mentally incapable, although the attorney can resign. There is no system to monitor the way the attorney carries out his or her duties, although in Ireland they are obliged to keep adequate accounts. In England and Wales, the Court of Protection has the power to supervise an attorney's actions, but only does so in exceptional circumstances, for example, when an allegation of financial impropriety has been made.[16] However, the donor can complain to the Public Trust Office or the Court of Protection, who can then decide whether the attorney should be kept on or replaced by a receiver, who is subject to greater control but can only deal with financial matters.

Under the German system, there is some control, in that the guardian has to obtain approval for certain decisions. In recognition of the severe consequences that the loss of a home can have on the person with dementia (from both an economic and a psychological point of view), special protective measures have been introduced. Furthermore, guardians have a legal responsibility towards the sufferer. Failure to carry out their duties, either wilfully or due to neglect, can result in legal action and possibly the obligation to pay compensation (this is also the case according to the Danish guardianship law). As a further safeguard, the guardianship must be terminated the moment that it is no longer necessary. In the case of dementia, this time is unlikely to come, but there is also a maximum period of five years, after which the guardianship must be renewed or cancelled. Again, this permits some measure of control.

The role of the patient in the decision-making process

Even when a person's mental capacity is greatly reduced and he/she can no longer make a decision alone, it is still possible in many cases to involve the person in the decision-making process. In the case of AD and certain related disorders, competence is not an all or nothing affair. Consequently, the preferences of a person who has been declared incompetent should, whenever possible, be taken into account by other people when making the decision. In some countries, legislation on guardianship stipulates that the person who is under guardianship should be consulted when decisions (especially important ones) are made.

According to Berghmans and Widdershoven, the following guidelines should be considered with regard to decision making and dementia.[17]

- The fact that a person has dementia does not necessarily mean they are to be considered incompetent and incapable of making decisions.

- Whether or not someone is considered incompetent depends on the type of decisions which have to be taken. A person with dementia can be perfectly capable of taking some decisions but incapable of taking others. Only when a person reaches the final stage of the disease is it acceptable to say that the person is totally incompetent.
- Decision-making capacity and competence can depend on matters such as the time of day or the mood of the person with dementia.

Consent to treatment and to participate in research

Situations can arise when it is impossible to obtain informed consent, but a decision must nevertheless be made, e.g. concerning residential care, the use of life-saving medication or techniques, participation in drug trials, etc. In many cases, a family member or guardian will consent on behalf of the person with dementia, but this is of course regulated by law, which differs according to the country. Furthermore, the person with dementia may not have an official guardian or relatives who can be consulted. However, in most countries if the person cannot consent and has no legal representative, the doctor can take the decision to give emergency treatment subject to certain conditions. In Denmark, doctors can also take decisions which are not related to urgent treatment in the absence of an official representative, but must obtain the approval of another health professional if the proposed treatment is not of a minor nature. Moreover, if the doctor feels that guardians have not used their power to consent in the best interests of the patient, he/she can take the appropriate action, provided that approval has been obtained from the relevant authorities.

Clark and Cantley pointed out some additional problems, which concern people with dementia making decisions related to their participation in research.[18]

- Who decides whether the person is competent?
- What should be done if the person's present decision is in total contradiction with his/her previous attitudes and stated beliefs?
- How might the existence of anxiety and depression affect decision making?
- How might the perceived power differential between researchers and the person with dementia affect the decision taken?

- Can the researcher be sure that the person has fully understood and will remember having made the decision?
- What provisions can be made for the person to withdraw from research (in view of his/her declining cognitive abilities)?

Advance directives

One possible solution is for the person with dementia to write an advance directive, a living will, in which he/she states future requirements with regard to care. Unfortunately, living wills are not legally binding in the majority of countries in Europe, although Article 9 of the Convention on Human Rights and Biomedicine states that the previously expressed wishes relating to a medical intervention by a patient, who is not at the time of the intervention in a state to express his or her wishes, shall be taken into account.[19]

In the United Kingdom, there is no legislation governing the use of advance directives but, according to a recent High Court ruling, advance directives made by mentally competent people about future treatment are legally binding.[20] In Switzerland, advance directives are now legally binding in five cantons. For example, in Geneva, health professionals are legally obliged to respect the wishes of a patient regarding decisions which relate to therapeutic treatment or care that the patient envisaged in his/her advance directive. This is even applicable in cases where the patient has refused life-saving treatment. For an advance directive to be valid, it must have been written before the person became incapable of discernment. This yet again emphasises the importance of an early diagnosis. The Dutch Medical Treatment Contract Act, which came into force in 1995, contains an article which addresses the issue of advance directives. It states that the doctor must comply with the apparent opinion of the patient expressed in writing while they are still capable of a reasonable assessment of their interests. However, the same article specifies that the doctor may deviate from this if he/she considers that there are good reasons for doing so. The Danish Law on Patients' Legal Status of 1998 contains a section on living wills. Such a will can be used to state preferences regarding resuscitation, and medical staff must consult a registry to check whether one has been made. It is legally binding if the patient is facing unavoidable death, but merely advisory in other cases.

In general, advance directives can include instructions relating not only to healthcare but also to non-medical issues such as the desire to remain at home for as long as possible, wishes related to religious beliefs, organ donation or agreement to take part in medical research. The right to refuse life-saving or sustaining treatment and to be allowed aggressive pain-killing treatment (even at the risk of hastening death) is a major concern for many people with dementia and can be linked to definable stages of the illness. A study carried out by Heap *et al.* in Great Britain, revealed that 86% of elderly patients would not want artificial ventilation if they were too confused to be safely left alone.[21] Furthermore, of 300 out-patients questioned, only 10% stated that they would definitely want cardiopulmonary resuscitation in case of cardiac arrest, should they be senile and no longer able to recognise familiar people.[21]

Even in countries where advance directives are not legally binding, they can be useful in helping doctors and family members to make a decision on behalf of the person with dementia when he/she is no longer competent. It is therefore important to work towards the acceptance of advance directives as legally binding documents, whilst at the same time devising guidelines to help people write them in such a way as to be sure that they will be interpreted in the intended way by those who eventually refer to them. As pointed out by Robertson,[20] patients need advice on the kind of terminology to use in order to express their wishes in a way which is neither too general nor too specific and which is most likely to lead to a uniform interpretation by doctors. This can perhaps be best achieved through discussion between the person with dementia, carers and doctors. Another approach is to provide guidelines for lawyers or others who may be involved in drawing up advance directives. Such guidelines were provided in a recent article in the internal newsletter of the public guardians – the legal representatives for patients in Austria.[22]

The issue of consent in the Convention on Human Rights and Biomedicine

The majority of EU member states signed the Convention on Human Rights and Biomedicine.[19] This convention deals specifically with the issue of consent, and Article 6 deals with the protection of people who are unable to give that consent. It states that:

- an intervention can only be carried out on a person who does not have the capacity to consent if the said intervention is for his or her direct benefit
- an intervention can only be carried out with the authorisation of his or her representative or an authority or a person or body provided for by law

- the individual concerned should, as far as possible, take part in the authorisation procedures
- the authorisation made on the person's behalf can be withdrawn at any time in the best interests of the person concerned.

With regard to people with a mental disorder, Article 7 states:

Subject to protective conditions prescribed by law, including supervisory, control and appeal procedures, a person who has a mental disorder of a serious nature may be subjected, without his or her consent, to an intervention aimed at treating his or her mental disorder only where, without such treatment, serious harm is likely to result to his or her health.

In addition to guidelines which are applicable for anyone participating in research, Article 17 of this Convention stipulates, with regard to people who are unable to consent, that:

- the results of the research must have the potential to produce real and direct benefit to the participant's health
- research of comparable effectiveness cannot be carried out on individuals capable of giving consent
- the necessary authorisation has been given specifically and in writing
- the person concerned does not object.

However, provided that the above additional conditions have been met, research which does not have a direct beneficial effect on the person's health can be carried out on people who are unable to consent if two conditions are fulfilled, namely:

- that the research has the aim of contributing, through significant improvement in the scientific understanding of the individual's condition, disease or disorder, to the ultimate attainment of results capable of conferring benefit on the person concerned or to other persons in the same age category or afflicted with the same disease or disorder or having the same condition
- that the research entails only minimal risk and minimal burden for the individual concerned.

The above article would presumably be applicable in the case of drug trials whereby the person with dementia could receive a placebo and not necessarily directly benefit from the research, even though the results of the research could benefit others in the future.

It is important to bear in mind that this convention is not legally binding and does not replace national legislation. It does, however, address the particular issue of consent to treatment and to participation in research in cases where the previous wishes of the person who is unable to consent are not known and there is no advance directive. Moreover, it may eventually serve as a guideline for future legislation on a national level.

Access to care and treatment

Entitlement to care across Europe

An individual is restricted in their request for a particular kind of care by the availability and possibility of obtaining such care in a particular country or region. Choice may be limited by a number of factors. The availability of care may not be uniform within a country. In addition, there may be costs involved or lengthy waiting lists. Some countries have specific legislation granting the right to appropriate treatment for people with dementia, whereas others have none which is specific to people with dementia. In some cases there is one overall law, whereas in others there are several laws which oblige different organisations to provide different forms of care.

In Portugal, for example, people with dementia are entitled to medical care on the same basis as other members of the population.[23] They are entitled to certain benefits on the basis of their age if over 65, but these benefits are no different from those available to other members of the population of the same age. This is similar to the situation in Austria, where people with dementia are entitled to receive the appropriate care and treatment, but only on the same basis as any other citizen. Again, they have no special entitlement solely on the grounds of the disease. In the Spanish Constitution, everyone has the same right to access to care but there is a special clause which stipulates that physically and mentally handicapped people should be given the specialised care that they require.

In Denmark, not only is there a lack of legislation which deals specifically with the entitlement of people with dementia to appropriate care, but the care of the elderly (including those with dementia) is dependent on policy decisions made by local councils.[24]

In the United Kingdom, people with dementia are entitled to social services under the Chronically Sick and Disabled Persons Act of 1970.

They are also entitled to benefit from residential accommodation according to the National Assistance Act of 1948 and care under the National Health Service (as are all citizens and residents).

In Sweden, all members of society are entitled to care. Responsibility for the care of the elderly rests with the State and is regulated by legislation. The Social Services Act of 1998 marked a transition of responsibility for the care of the elderly (including those with dementia) from county councils to municipalities.[25] This Act granted people the right to demand help and services which, if not provided, could justify an appeal.

The availability of treatment across Europe

Support and assistance for carers is important in view of the fact that the vast majority of people with dementia throughout Europe are cared for at home. It is also important to bear in mind that even when legislation exists, this does not automatically mean that the person with dementia will benefit from the services or care. In Luxembourg, for example, places in day centres are limited and there is an average waiting period of three years for a place in a home.[26] Consequently, a large number of people suffering from AD continue to be cared for at home.

The availability and price of drugs varies from one country in Europe to the next. Prescription patterns also vary between and within countries. In the United Kingdom, for example, different health authorities have different policies on the prescription of particular drugs within the National Health Service. Consequently, although general practitioners are free to prescribe any available drug, they may be influenced in the extent that they prescribe it and some patients may have to pay more to obtain it.[27]

Some drugs, such as Aricept and Exelon (which are used in the treatment of AD in the early to mid-stages), have been approved by the European Commission for all countries in Europe, although they are not yet available in some. A questionnaire sent to different Alzheimer's associations in Europe at the beginning of 1998 revealed that three drugs, Cognex, Aricept and Exelon, were available in only four countries (Finland, France, Germany and Sweden), five countries had two of these drugs and seven had only one. There is, however, no evidence of any effect in the severe stage of the disease and the long-term effects of the new drugs are not known.[28]

The increase in accurate and up-to-date information on AD, particularly on the Internet, has resulted in a certain degree of frustration with regard to the availability of drugs. Alzheimer Europe regularly receives emails from individuals in countries where a particular drug is not available, hoping to obtain information on how to obtain it from another country. This situation will eventually be partly resolved when Aricept and Exelon are available in all countries. In addition, there are a number of drugs under development, some of which are awaiting approval. Yet other drugs, such as Cognex, did not benefit from authorisation on a European level and are not scheduled to become available in all countries. Others are awaiting approval in one or more European countries.

Legal obligation for families to provide care

Throughout Europe, the majority of people suffering from AD are cared for at home. In some countries, caring for a frail or dependent family member is actually an obligation for parents, children or the extended family, whereas in others it is not. In yet other countries, the state has clearly defined obligations concerning the provision of care and the family has few obligations. In a recent study carried out by Miller and Warman, the respective role of the family and the state was analysed for different countries in Europe.[29] Four clear categories emerged concerning the legal obligation to provide care (*see* Figure 3.1).

Group 1 comprises three southern member states (Italy, Spain and Portugal) in which members of the extended family have legal obligations

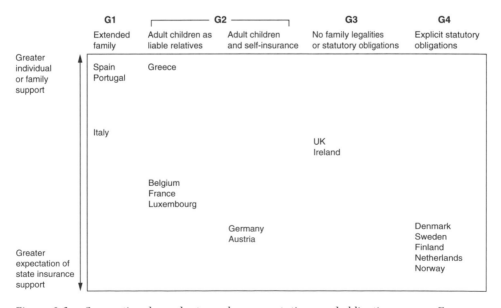

Figure 3.1: Supporting dependent people – expectations and obligations across Europe.

to provide financial support to dependent relatives. Since the state has little responsibility to support individuals, those needing assistance with care have to pay for it themselves. If this is not possible, family members are obliged either to provide the care themselves or to fund it.

Group 2 comprises Austria, Germany, Belgium, France, Luxembourg and Greece. Maintenance responsibilities are limited to adult children, who are deemed to be 'liable relatives' and may be asked to pay for their parents' support. The state has powers to reclaim financial benefits from adult children.

The statutory duties have recently been further modified in Austria and Germany, where all adults are now required to contribute to an insurance fund for their own future care. In Germany, for example, the *Pflegeversicherung* is a universal scheme which funds, through compulsory contributions, both residential and domiciliary care for older people. Payments can be made for family care, which may provide an incentive to keep an elderly relative at home. Three levels of severity of disability determine the amount of financial support, but it has been suggested that the need for support among people with dementia has been underestimated.

In Group 3, containing Ireland and the United Kingdom, there are neither formal legal obligations upon families to support older people, nor clear statutory responsibilities towards individuals in need of support. This situation is surprising given the recognition in the UK of the crucial role of family carers, but less so with a legal system based on the force of eligibility criteria rather than rights. This will probably change with the advance of the European human rights legislation.

The five countries that make up Group 4 (Denmark, Sweden, Finland, the Netherlands and Norway) have explicit statutory obligations towards vulnerable people. Individuals who are unable to meet the costs of their own residential care or domiciliary services are entitled to financial support from government funds. In Sweden and Norway, wages may also be paid to relatives who provide care to disabled family members.

The different approaches to the relative involvement of the state and the family in the provision of care may result from an interaction between historical, social, cultural, political and economic factors. Access to care, treatment and medication continues to be provided in a non-uniform manner across Europe. Government policy decisions continue to determine the availability of care and treatment, as well as entitlement to it. Other factors such as geographical location, finances, the availability of information and referral or diagnostic procedures also play a role.

Consequences of dementia for carers and families

In the southern countries where families are legally bound to care for their relatives with dementia, there are few, if any, financial incentives. The obligation is in fact closely linked to the cultural sense of duty between family members. This contrasts with other countries where, even though the state is responsible for care to a greater or lesser extent, family members who provide care are eligible in certain circumstances for financial benefits and support.

In Luxembourg, for example, carers are entitled to tax exemptions, a fixed sum care allowance (amounting to approximately euro 500) and an allowance towards the cost of home help. The allowance towards the cost of home help, which consists of a tax exemption of approximately euro 600, can only be granted if the person hired is declared to the Social Services Department. It is interesting to note that the hired person can be a brother or sister but not a son, daughter, father or mother. This seems to reflect the attitude that the act of caring is considered to be a duty when carried out by certain relatives. Indeed the very people who are excluded from receiving such support form a large proportion of those who throughout Europe care for people suffering from AD, i.e. daughters and (in the case of younger sufferers) close relatives, which could include parents. However, in Luxembourg, the situation is gradually changing as the new care insurance is slowly implemented.

In the United Kingdom, the invalid care allowance can be paid to carers regardless of their relationship to the person they are caring for, provided that they do not earn more than a particular fixed amount per week. However, this allowance can only be paid to carers of people who are already receiving an attendance or disability living allowance.

As pointed out by Levi, the socio-economic consequences of AD vary, depending on its severity, from onset through to the later stages.[30] However, the burden of caring may be increased as a result of other factors such as the competing demands of paid employment, age, personal health or the double burden of caring for both younger and older relatives.

In many countries, a carer may become the official guardian of a person with dementia, but in many cases the carers of people with dementia are not officially declared or legally recognised. This state of affairs can be reflected in a lack of due consideration for their own personal needs arising as a result of their role.

Abuse, safety and discrimination

Elder abuse

The combined problem of dementia and abuse

There are many different forms of elder abuse which take place in both the home and the institutional setting, including physical and verbal abuse, as well as neglect. Abuse can take the form of excessive medication, e.g. sedation which is administered with the aim of controlling socially disruptive or deviant behaviour rather than to calm the person with dementia. A Swedish study revealed that 44% of patients in nursing homes were taking medication they did not need. The forcing of fluid or food on the person with dementia (e.g. feeding by tube) and the systematic enforcement of hygienic measures such as washing and dressing can also be construed as abuse. Finally, there is psychological abuse. This could, for example, take the form of emotional blackmail, threats, ridicule or talking down to the person with dementia as if they were a child.

People with dementia often find themselves in a situation of dependency on the person who assures their care. This can make it difficult for them to obtain help in cases of abuse, particularly if they also have limited contact with the outside world. Due to the decline of cognitive abilities – a common feature of dementia – the person who is in an abusive situation may be unaware of the fact or unable to communicate the problem. Furthermore, certain forms of abuse such as neglect, verbal abuse and chemical restraint may not be immediately obvious to visiting outsiders. In residential or day care, people with dementia may fear retaliation or punitive measures from their abusers. Carers might also fear retaliation against their relative, should they complain to professional carers.

Finally, there is the issue of self-neglect, whereby a person with dementia may be living alone in conditions of squalor, lacking in hygiene, adequate nutrition and human contact. Such conditions can exacerbate their condition.

Research into the frequency of abuse and possible contributing factors

There is no shortage of research which bears testimony to the practice of elder abuse. A study carried out in the Netherlands,[31] revealed high levels of verbal aggression (30% of carers), as well as physical aggression (10% of carers). In the UK, a study carried out by Cooney and Mortimer revealed that 55% of people who responded admitted having abused the person with dementia for whom they were caring, with verbal abuse being most common.[32] According to Paveza *et al.*, a person with AD is at least twice as likely to suffer from physical abuse as an elderly person who does not have it.[33]

There are several possible causes for the high frequency of abuse on the elderly with dementia. Pillemer and Suiter found that the violence tended to be related to disruptive behaviour by the person with dementia and the fact of living with a carer (as tension and conflict are perhaps more difficult to avoid due to the close proximity).[34] In a study carried out by Podnieks in Canada, it was revealed that 56% of abusive caregivers were suffering from psychiatric or emotional problems and that 70% reported serious problems with their physical health.[35] Nevertheless, it is most likely that a combination of factors is involved.

Restraint/protective measures

Carers, both at home and in the residential setting, often consider it necessary to restrict the free movement of people with dementia. Apart from chemical forms of restraint, leather straps are sometimes used to confine a person with dementia to a bed, chair or commode. This not only deprives the person of their freedom, but can also have severe consequences for health and well-being, creating fear, frustration and humiliation, causing pressure sores and contributing to accidents. The use of restrictive measures can also violate the dignity of a person with dementia, as it can affect a person's sense of self and self-esteem. The use of physical forms of restraint can be classed as abusive but is often justified on the grounds that it protects the person with dementia from coming to any harm or harming others. However, research has shown that there is no scientific evidence to prove that restraint guarantees the patient's safety, and some reports have even concluded that protective measures can sometimes result in serious harm to the patient.

Berghmans and Widdershoven also drew up the following list of questions which they felt should be answered whenever the use of protective measures is considered.[17]

1 What is the background to the problem behaviour of the person with dementia?
2 Why is the use of protective measures contemplated?
3 To what extent does the anxiety of staff and other carers play a role?
4 Are all the people concerned sufficiently involved in the decision-making process?
5 Have alternative, less restrictive courses of action been examined?
6 Is the reason for the use of a protective measure serious enough?

7   Does the intervention have a positive risk–benefit ratio?
8   Is the legal position of the person with dementia sufficiently guaranteed?
9   Is informed consent given by the patient or his/her representative?
10 Is regular evaluation of the need and justification for (continuation of) the restraint measure provided for?
11 Has any assistance necessary for the patient been considered?

They further propose that in view of the drastic nature of protective measures, a clear policy should be formulated by institutions. This should include a statement of values and principles applied to specific situations and examples of criteria upon which to base a decision on the possible use of such measures.

Legislation relating to abuse

Legislation across Europe addresses the issue of abuse in its various forms, i.e. restraint, exploitation, abuse, abandonment and neglect, although not always with specific regard to dementia. Forced internment tends to be covered by laws relating to psychiatric internment.

With regard to measures which restrain or restrict the freedom of movement of a person under guardianship (including the use of straps, locked doors and medication), under the German system, the guardian must obtain permission from the appropriate court or, in case of emergency, must obtain approval immediately afterwards.

In Spain, exploitation, abuse and abandonment of a person with dementia can give rise to both criminal and civil liability.[12] This could involve the obligation to give compensation for damages to the person and the family of those with dementia. If the person who is responsible works for the administration, administrative liability may also apply, e.g. fines, closing orders, etc. However, this depends on the abuse being reported.

In the United Kingdom, a report by the Law Commission recommended that where a local authority has reason to believe that a vulnerable person in their area is suffering or likely to suffer significant harm or serious exploitation, they shall make such enquiries as they consider necessary to enable them to decide:

•   whether the person is in fact suffering or likely to suffer such harm or exploitation, and if so
•   whether community care services should be provided or arranged or other actions taken to protect the person from such harm or exploitation.

Legislation relating to forced internment

In general, people with dementia can be interned if they constitute a danger to themselves and/or others or if they are in need of medical care. Normally, the period is either for a specific length of time, which can be extended, or, in the case of Germany, until the conditions which led to it are no longer valid. In the United Kingdom, the suspicion of various forms of abuse and neglect can also be used as a justification for emergency action.

Table 3.1 provides an example of the different conditions which may justify internment in a number of countries and which could in certain cases apply to a person suffering from dementia.

From these examples, two main issues emerge: protection of oneself and others; and the need for treatment. However, before internment can occur, numerous other conditions must be fulfilled, such as medical examinations and reports. The European Council in 1983 recommended that a person should only be interned if they present a grave danger to themselves or others or if their condition would deteriorate in the absence of placement.[36] Once confined, the person's liberty should be restricted only to the extent necessary. This is not covered in much of the legislation. Moreover, at the 3rd European Conference of Family Law, organised by the Council of Europe in 1995, concern was expressed that people lacking full mental capacity were being unnecessarily institutionalised by family members, friends or government officials using vague and overly broad legislative mandates. The fear was expressed that the criterion of risk to self or others is difficult to evaluate. On the other hand, attempts to reduce involuntary detention have resulted in reducing access to treatment in some countries.[37]

Clearly, a balance is necessary between the need to provide care and the wish not to unnecessarily restrict liberty. Possible solutions to the problem of handling abuse and neglect, both within institutions and in the home, include the following: the setting up of a system, such as the Confidential Doctors' Offices, which have been effective in the Netherlands in tackling the problems of child abuse and neglect; and/or the appointment of an ombudsman or commissioner to protect the interests of people with dementia.

Preventing the person with dementia from driving

The risks involved

As cognitive abilities deteriorate, the ability to drive gradually declines, and this results in the individual becoming a potential danger to both self

Table 3.1: Justification for internment for mental disorder in selected European countries

Country	Conditions for forced internment (any can apply)
France	1 If a person suffering from a mental disorder is unable to consent. 2 His/her condition demands immediate treatment combined with constant observation in a hospital setting.
Germany	1 If, due to the fact that the person is suffering from a mental illness or mental handicap, there is a danger that he/she will kill him/herself or cause considerable damage to his/her own health; or 2 If it is necessary to carry out a medical examination or treatment which cannot otherwise be carried out without the person being committed and due to the nature of the illness the person does not recognise the necessity for commitment or cannot act in accordance with this understanding.
Luxembourg	People suffering from mental disorders may be placed in a closed psychiatric establishment or department only if serious mental disorder makes them a danger to themselves or others (if the person can be cared for at home, 'home confinement' is possible).
Netherlands	1 If, as a result of a disturbance of mental capacity (due to pathological development of mental capacity or a mental illness), the person constitutes a danger to him/herself; and 2 If the danger cannot be averted by the intervention of persons or institutions other than a psychiatric hospital and the person does not consent to being admitted.
Portugal	1 If a person, suffering from a serious mental illness, as a result of the illness, threatens the judicial property of significant value, either belonging to him/herself or to others, of a personal or equity nature, and refuses to submit him/herself to the necessary medical treatment. 2 If a person suffering from a serious mental illness, does not possess the necessary judgement to evaluate the meaning and extent of consent, and the absence of treatment is causing acute deterioration to his/her state.
United Kingdom	1 If a person is suffering from mental illness, severe mental impairment, psychopathic disorder or mental impairment and this mental disorder is of a nature or degree which makes it appropriate for him/her to receive medical treatment in a hospital; and 2 In the case of psychopathic disorder or mental impairment, such treatment is likely to alleviate or prevent a deterioration of his/her condition; and 3 It is necessary for the health and safety of the patient or for the protection of other persons that he/she should receive such treatment and it cannot be provided unless he/she is detained.

and others. Several studies have estimated that the probability of a crash among drivers with dementia is at least twice as high than for other drivers. Studies by Drachman and Swearer[38] and Waller et al.[39] led to the conclusion that crashes involving people with dementia are not evenly distributed over the disease's duration, in that drivers with AD do not tend to pose a risk during the first three years. These findings were not backed up by earlier studies carried out by Friedland et al., who found no correlation between the number of accidents and duration of the dementia.[40] Nevertheless, there is a general consensus that drivers with dementia have a higher risk of crashes than do drivers from the older population in general.

If the dementia sufferer is aware of the diagnosis, they may stop driving as soon as difficulties arise. However, as the disease progresses, insight may also deteriorate and the person may have difficulty in dealing with loss of the ability to drive, which for many people is symbolic of independence and may be their only way of getting about. If relatives are informed of the diagnosis, they may have to try to stop the person from driving, and this is not always an easy task. Unfortunately, someone who has been given legal responsibility for the welfare of the person with dementia might not necessarily be able to prevent them from driving, unless it is possible actually to dispose of the car. Carers faced with this situation often have to devise means of preventing the person from driving when they refuse to listen, e.g. removing the distributor cap, parking the car away from the house, hiding the keys, or creating a distraction.

Provisions and conditions for the withdrawal of a driving licence

In certain countries, provisions are made to withdraw driving licences from people who are no longer in a fit condition to drive. In the United Kingdom, for example, anyone who is affected by a medical condition that impairs their ability to drive is obliged to inform the Driver and Vehicle Licensing Agency (DVLA). A doctor or relative can also inform the DVLA on behalf of the person with dementia. The DVLA then contacts the doctor, and after that, the patient. In Sweden, doctors are obliged to report patients who are obviously unfit to drive, although this does not always happen. There are, however, very few guidelines concerning the assessment of drivers with dementia. In Sweden, licences are granted for life. The renewal procedure is a mere formality, which does not necessitate a medical examination or any kind of test. For this reason, age-related decline or illnesses may go unnoticed at the time of renewal.

Under Austrian law, a driving licence can be withdrawn on the grounds of physical and/or mental factors which interfere with the ability to drive, rather than merely due to a diagnosis of dementia. Driving can be restricted locally or temporarily.[41] This means that a person could, for example, be allowed to drive only in a particular village or neighbourhood and only during the day.

In France, even if a doctor becomes aware that a patient is unfit to drive, they can only recommend to the patient that the individual give up driving. The potential danger to the patient and others is not sufficient justification to report the matter to the administrative authorities. There is a clear conflict between the doctor's obligation to respect the principle of confidentiality and the need to protect the patient and other people from the consequences of dementia.

In Scotland, medical ethics also dictate that the relationship between the patient and the doctor remains confidential, but this obligation is not legally binding. Although a doctor could be prosecuted for breach of confidence, they could, in theory, justify disclosure of information to authorities or another person if it were considered to be necessary in the public interest.[42] This would presumably cover the issue of unfitness to drive.

In Sweden, concern has been expressed that the relationship between doctor and patient could be threatened by the practice of reporting to the authorities in cases of unfitness to drive or the automatic withdrawal of licences when dementia is diagnosed. Nevertheless, a consensus statement on dementia and driving, which resulted from a meeting held under the auspices of the Swedish Road Administration, stressed the important role of the doctor in ensuring the safety of patients and the general public. In this statement the following proposals were made.

- *A routine investigation should be carried out by the family physician.* Whenever an elderly patient comes to the physician for a consultation, the physician should inquire whether he or she is driving. If that should be the case, the physician should investigate whether the patient is suffering from possible cognitive impairment. If impairment is suspected, the patient should be examined on more than one occasion in order to determine the level and degree of impairment (e.g. visiospatial skills, attention, memory, judgement).
- *Background information and collateral reports should be obtained* (e.g. information on activities for daily living (ADL) functions and on the patient's past driving ability should be obtained from relatives). ADLs and independent activities for daily living (IADLs) (shopping, using public transport and handling finances) are considered to be better indicators of driving ability than cognitive tests.
- *The physician should report a potential dangerous driver to the authorities and should also inform the patient.* This should be documented in the medical record and given to the patient in writing, as well as to the carer if necessary. In recognition of the fact that the onset of

dementia can be gradual, if a patient is cognitively impaired but still capable of driving, the physician should inform the patient and their relatives of the increased risk of crashes among cognitively impaired drivers, and advise about any possible adaptive driving strategies.

In 1998 a series of forums took place in different regions of France. Participants – who were all geriatricians, neurologists, GPs and psychiatrists – discussed a number of different issues, one of which was driving and legal protective measures. Several possible solutions were proposed, which can be summarised as follows:

- jobs should be created for young people that would consist in driving people with dementia around
- the doctor should evaluate the patient and advise them, as well as the family, orally but also in writing on any reservations with regard to driving
- a score of 18 on the Mini-mental State (MMS) should lead to a restriction being imposed on the person with dementia to drive only if accompanied – this did not meet with unanimity from the group
- the person should be allowed to drive in limited areas, on familiar roads and only if accompanied by someone who knows the road.

The issue of driving is just one example of a problem which arises when it is necessary to strike a balance between the need to protect the individual and the general public. It is further complicated by the fact that the relationship between the doctor and the patient is of a confidential nature, but the doctor may, in many cases, be the only person who is sufficiently aware of the patient's condition, and hence in a position to take the appropriate action. Any legislation which aims to enforce reporting by doctors could jeopardise the doctor–patient relationship and possibly prevent people from consulting doctors in the case of problems which they suspect to be due to dementia. Compulsory medical visits for licence holders above a particular age might reduce this problem and lead to the early detection of undiagnosed cases of dementia as well as improving road safety. Nevertheless, this would necessitate the development of effective methods of testing which would enable the detection of problems related to driving, whilst not penalising older people who are still able to drive.

Consequences of dementia for sufferers in paid employment

People with dementia who are still in paid employment may experience difficulties continuing their work. Symptoms such as poor concentration, problems with attention and abstract reasoning, may lead them to a gradual deterioration in the quality of their work and perhaps serious mistakes. As they are likely to be under 65, it is possible that it could take some time before a diagnosis of dementia is obtained, as numerous other possibilities would be considered. Many general practitioners have very little experience of early onset dementia and may even rule out the possibility. The symptoms may be confused with other disorders and they might think that the problem is due to the menopause, depression or migraine, or even drug misuse.

It would, however, be preferable for someone with dementia to obtain a diagnosis before the situation deteriorated to such an extent that they were dismissed, given that this could affect pension rights and the possibility of obtaining benefits. Dementia can also result in a double loss of income, as a relative of the sufferer may also have to leave their job in order to ensure appropriate care. This can have disastrous consequences, particularly on younger sufferers who have not finished paying off a mortgage or who have other financial obligations.

Genetic testing and insurance companies

Testing for AD

It is now known that three genes play a role in early onset of familial AD. These are the amyloid precursor protein (APP) gene on chromosome 21, the presenilin-1 (PS-1) gene on chromosome 14 and the presenilin-2 (PS-2) gene on chromosome 1.[43] For early onset familial AD, both predictive and diagnostic testing is possible. With the former, it is possible to detect which individuals will eventually develop the inherited condition, whereas the latter can be used to confirm a diagnosis that has already been made. In all cases, it is preferable that testing is preceded, accompanied and followed by comprehensive counselling.

In recent years, the identification of a gene on chromosome 19, responsible for the production of a protein called apolipoprotein E (ApoE), has enabled researchers to identify people who are more at risk of developing AD than others. There are three main variants of this protein: E2, E3 and E4. Although uncommon, E4 increases the likelihood of a person developing AD, but does not cause the disease. E2, on the other hand, probably decreases the risk or is protective. It is important to note that many people with AD do not have E4 and many who do have E4, do not develop the disease. Furthermore, despite the fact that there is no precedent for this kind of testing and even though people with this protein will not all develop the disease, it is being offered by at least one commercial testing facility in the United States and another in Europe.

Safeguarding the interests of the person tested

Apart from the possibly unjustified fear or even relief that such testing might produce in individuals, as well as the consequences for a person's family, there are other potential dangers, for example, the issue of confidentiality. The recording of data and its transmission to third parties threatens the relationship between doctor and patient, which is based on professional secrecy and confidentiality.

However, the establishment of epidemiological registers is a common practice in many public health authorities and one which allows them to plan healthcare needs and define the groups which are most at risk. Databases containing medical information can be accessed by medical researchers and professionals. One solution to this problem would be to have anonymous registers, as is the case in France, and also to grant people the right to refuse the transmission of any information to third parties, even that which is registered anonymously.

The Council of Europe has laid down guidelines.[44] The following points are relevant.

- Genetic tests may only be carried out on the authority of a duly qualified physician (Principle 2).
- Any genetic testing and screening procedure should be accompanied by appropriate counselling, both before and after the procedure (Principle 3).
- The testing of persons suffering from mental disorders should be subject to special safeguards (Principle 5).
- The consent of the person to be tested should be obtained, except where national law provides otherwise (Principle 5).
- In genetic screening and testing or associated genetic counselling, personal data may be collected, processed and stored only for the purposes of healthcare, diagnosis and disease prevention, and for research closely related to these matters (Principle 8).
- Persons handling genetic information should be bound by professional rules of conduct and rules laid down by national legislation aimed at preventing the misuse of such information and in particular by the duty to observe strict confidentiality. Personal information obtained by genetic testing is protected on the same basis as other medical data by the rules of medical data protection. However, in the case of a severe genetic risk for other family members, consideration should be given, in accordance with national legislation and professional rules of conduct, to informing family members about matters relevant to their health or that of their future children (Principle 9).

- Samples collected for a specific medical or scientific purpose may not, without permission of the persons concerned or the persons legally entitled to give permission on their behalf, be used in ways which could be harmful to the persons concerned. The use of genetic data for population and similar studies has to respect rules governing data protection, and in particular concerning anonymity and confidentiality. The same applies to the publishing of such data (Principle 13).

Whilst this sets out general guidelines for carrying out genetic testing, it is not specific to susceptibility testing for AD. A consensus statement on predictive testing for AD issued by the medical and scientific advisory committee of Alzheimer's Disease International expressed concern over the use of presymptomatic testing. They concluded that apart from a few rare families with early onset familial AD associated with the APP mutations, the time for presymptomatic predictive testing for AD in general had not yet arrived.

Interest in genetic testing from insurance companies

There is considerable interest in such testing from insurance companies. In fact, insurers had expressed interest in the issue of genetic testing in relation to insurance as early as 1935 on the occasion of the International Congress of Life Assurance Medicine, when Fischer stated that:

> . . . linkage groups should be sorted out, in order to trace the inheritance and predict the occurrence of other factors of greater individual importance, such as those producing insanity, various forms of mental deficiency and other transmissible diseases.[45]

As pointed out by Ewald of the French Federation of Insurance Societies, the notion of insurance is linked with that of risk and uncertainty, but strictly speaking, insurance is impossible if the risk has already occurred or is certain to occur in the future.[46] Furthermore, the insurer must have some notion of the probability of a risk and its gravity in order to be able to charge the correct price for it according to its probability. Insurers may be knowledgeable about probabilities based on populations, but individuals may have personal knowledge about their own risk. Doctors may also have such information, but are bound by laws on medical secrecy (which in France are absolute). The onus is consequently on the individual to disclose information about themselves, failure to do so resulting in the nullification of the contract. In France, the insurer can ask questions or give the individual a questionnaire.

If a medical examination is required, it must be carried out by a doctor who would also be bound by secrecy laws. This means that they would not have the right to give the information to the insurer, even if employed by the organisation, but would give an opinion on the probability of the risk. Consequently the individual may therefore find themselves discriminated against on the basis of their genes, regardless of the fact that they may never develop the disease. Alzheimer's Disease International considers the sensitivity and specificity rates for the ApoE4 test to be too low to be used as a diagnostic test, a view which is echoed in the Report *Mental disorders and genetics: the ethical context* by the UK Nuffield Council of Bioethics.[47]

Possible solutions

According to Article 6 of the 1997 Universal Declaration on the Human Genome and Human Rights:

> *No one shall be subjected to discrimination based on genetic characteristics that is intended to infringe or has the effect of infringing human rights, fundamental freedoms and human dignity.*

Discrimination against individuals on the grounds of knowledge gained from genetic testing could eventually result in fewer people having recourse to it.

One solution used by insurance companies in the Netherlands was to agree not to require genetic testing for insurance sums below 200 000 Florins.[48] In the United Kingdom, the Human Genetics Advisory Commission stated that the information linking genetics and multifactorial disease was at too early a stage to make sound assessments of added risk. They also recommended that although it might be possible to legislate against any requirement to disclose genetic test results, it would be preferable to agree on a moratorium, with a mechanism for making specific exceptions in view of the rapidly changing advances in the field. This recommendation was partly based on the view that more research was needed into the actuarial implications of genetic research. Nevertheless, the Alzheimer's Society (UK) recently felt obliged to transfer its insurance business from a particular insurance company which could not ensure that it would not discriminate against people with dementia applying for long-term insurance.[49]

Conclusions

As can be seen from the first section of this chapter, there is a growing awareness and recognition that people with dementia have rights, in particular the right to self-determination, and that this does not stop when a diagnosis of dementia is made. This is accompanied by a gradual move away from a paternalistic approach. Clearly, an appropriate balance must be struck between freedom and protection; and this is reflected in the most recently adopted or amended laws on guardianship and in the recommendations on principles concerning the legal protection of incapable adults produced by the Council of Europe in 1999.[50]

The extremely important role of informal carers remains unclear, and legal recognition under-developed. Campaigning groups such as Alzheimer Europe and its member organisations are campaigning for recognition of the legal status of principal care-givers and their inclusion in decisions concerning the provision of care and the development of appropriate services.

The second section of this chapter outlined the difficulties in ensuring that people with dementia are not mistreated, endangered or discriminated against in view of their particularly vulnerable position. A similar need to strike a balance is again required, this time between self-determination and protection, although there is the additional question of the necessity to also take into consideration the needs of other people (as in the case of driving) and the interests of other parties (such as insurance companies).

References

1   Downs M and Rae C (1996) *General practitioners' approach to establishing and communicating a diagnosis of dementia.* Annual Conference of the British Society of Gerontology, University of Liverpool.

2   Tiraboschi P, Moleri M, Defanti CA, Moretti C and Siegler M (1996) *Would physicians tell patients with Alzheimer's disease their diagnosis? Would they inform at risk persons if a genetic test became available?* Paper presented at the Alzheimer's Disease International Conference, Jerusalem.

3   Heal HC and Husband HJ (1998) Disclosing a diagnosis of dementia: is age a factor? *Aging and Mental Health.* 2(2): 144–50.

4   Novak DH *et al.* (1997) Changes in physicians' attitudes toward telling the cancer patient. *JAMA.* 241: 897–900.

5   Byrne EJ (1987) Reversible dementias. *Int J Ger Psych.* 6: 199–208.

6   Homer AC, Hanovar M, Lastos PL *et al.* (1988) Diagnosing dementia, do we always get it right? *BMJ.* 297: 894–6.

7   Erde EL, Nadal EC and Scholl TO (1988) On truth telling and the diagnosis of Alzheimer's disease. *J Fam Pract.* 26: 401–6.

8 Maguire CP, Kirby M, Coen R *et al.* (1996) Family members' attitudes toward telling the patient with Alzheimer's disease their diagnosis, *BMJ.*
313: 529–30.

9 *The Patient's Charter: a charter for health, 1991* (National Health Service) –
Scotland.

10 *The Charter of the Hospitalised Patient, 1990* – France.

11 *Civil Code, art. 501* – France.

12 *Article 215 to 306* of the *Civil Code* – Spain.

13 *Guardianship Law (Betreuungsgesetz) 1992.*

14 *The Guardianship Act, 1997.*

15 Martinez Montauti J (1995) *Medical treatment of incapacitated and other vulnerable adults and non-therapeutic research on these persons, including proper
safeguards of their best interests.* Proceedings of the 3rd European Conference
on Family Law organised by the Council of Europe in Cádiz, Spain.

16 Langan J and Means R (1996) Financial management and elderly people with
dementia in the UK: as much a question of confusion as abuse? *Ageing and
Society.* **16**: 287–314.

17 Berghmans RLP and Widdershoven GAM (1997) *Ethics in Dementia Care:
a booklet for professional carers.* Instituut voor Gezondheidsethiek, Maastricht.

18 Clark C and Cantley C (1998) Workshop entitled *The Ethics of conducting
research about and with people with dementia.* Dementia Care 98, 2 July 1998,
University of Loughborough.

19 Council of Europe (1997) *Convention for the Protection of Human Rights and
Dignity of the Human Being with regard to the Application of Biology and Medicine.*
Council of Europe, Strasbourg.

20 Robertson GS (1995) Making an advance directive. *BMJ.* **310**: 236–9.

21 Heap MJ, Munglani R, Klinck JR and Males AG (1993) Elderly patients' preferences concerning life support treatment. *Anaesthesia.* **48**: 1027–33.

22 Wagner M (1998) Die Patientenverfügung – Das psychiatrische Testament
als Schritt in Richtung Selbstbestimmung (Advance directives – the living
will as a step in the direction of self-determination). In: *Nachrichten aus
dem Rechtsreferat.* Verein für Sachwalterschaft und Patientenanwaltschaft,
Vienna.

23 Robusto-Leitao O and Pilao C (1998) *Transnational Analysis of the Socio-
economic Impact of Alzheimer's Disease in the European Union: the Portuguese case.*
London School of Economics, London.

24 Knudsen JL (1998) *Transnational Analysis of the Socio-economic Impact of
Alzheimer's Disease in the European Union: the Danish case.* London School of
Economics, London.

25   Social Services Act (SFS 1980:620/1998:855) 1998.

26   Goetschalckx C (1997) *European Transnational Alzheimer Study, National Report, Luxembourg*. Welsh Institute for Health and Social Care, University of Glamorgan.

27   Fearnley K (1999) Personal Communication.

28   Wimo A (1998) Dementia care: issues for European healthcare systems. *Eurohealth*. **4**(3).

29   Miller J and Warman A (1996) *Family Obligations in Europe*. London Family Studies Centre, London.

30   Levi L (1997) *Social and Economic Cost Calculation of AD and AD care*. EACH Report (WP4), Brussels.

31   Penhale B and Kingston P (1997) Elder abuse, mental health and later life: steps towards an understanding. *Aging and Mental Health*. **1**(4): 296–304.

32   Cooney C and Mortimer A (1995) Elder abuse and dementia. *Int J Soc Psych*. **41**: 276–83.

33   Paveza GJ, Cohen D, Eisdorfer C *et al.* (1992) Severe family violence and Alzheimer's disease: prevalence and risk factors. *Gerontologist*. **32**(4): 493–7.

34   Pillemer K and Suiter J (1992) Violence and violent feelings: What causes them among family caregivers? *J Gerontol*. **47**(4): 165–72.

35   Podnieks E (1990) National survey on abuse of the elderly in Canada. *J Elder Abuse Neglect*. **4**: 55–8.

36   Council of Europe (1983) *Recommendation (83) 2*. Committee of Ministers to Member States concerning the Legal Protection of Persons Suffering from Mental Disorder placed as Involuntary Patients. Council of Europe, Strasbourg.

37   Shelton D (1995) *Human rights of the incapacitated and other vulnerable adults*. Proceedings of the 3rd European Conference on Family Law organised by the Council of Europe in Cádiz, Spain.

38   Drachman DA and Swearer J (1993) Driving and Alzheimer's disease: the risk of crashes. *Neurology*. **43**: 2448–56.

39   Waller PF, Trobe JD and Olson PL (1993) *Crash characteristics associated with early Alzheimer's disease*. Presented at the 37th annual meeting of the Association for the Advancement of Automobile Medicine, November 4–6, San Antonio, Texas.

40   Friedland RP, Koss E, Kumar A *et al.* (1988) Motor vehicle crashes in dementia of the Alzheimer type. *Ann Neurol*. **24**: 782–6.

41   Jaquemar S (1998) (Rapporteur of Law Affairs of the Verein für Sachwalterschaft und Patientenanwaltschaft) Letter of 1/10/1998 – private communication.

42 Fearnley K, McLennan J and Weaks D (1997) *The Right to Know: sharing the diagnosis of dementia*. Alzheimer Scotland – Action on Dementia, Edinburgh.

43 Alzheimer's Disease International (1998) *Alzheimer's Disease and Genetics*. ADI, London.

44 Council of Europe (1992) *Recommendation (92) 3*. Committee of Ministers to Member States concerning Genetic Testing and Screening of Europe. Council of Europe, Strasbourg.

45 Nuffield Council on Bioethics (1993) *Genetic Screening Ethical Issues*. Nuffield Council on Bioethics, London.

46 Ewald F (1993) Comments made at the *Confidentiality issues in medical genetics* discussion. 2nd Symposium of the Council of Europe on Bioethics, Strasbourg.

47 Nuffield Council on Bioethics (1998) *Mental Disorders and Genetics: the ethical context*. Nuffield Council on Bioethics, London.

48 De Wachter MAM and van Luijk HJL (1993) Genetic information and health, life and disability insurance. In: H Haker, R Hearn and K Steigleder (eds) *Ethics of Human Genome Analysis*: European perspectives. Attempto Verlag, Tübingen.

49 Alzheimer's Disease Society (1997) *Newsletter*. **June**.

50 Council of Europe (1999) *Recommendation No R (99) 4*. Committee of Ministers to Member States on Principles Concerning the Legal Protection of Incapable Adults. Council of Europe, Strasbourg.

4

Carer burden: the difficulties and rewards of care-giving

Joanna Murray and David McDaid

Introduction

This chapter is concerned with the informal care of people with Alzheimer's disease (AD), provided mainly by unpaid family members, together with the variety of formal support they receive. In considering the balance of care within member states, two areas of research can be drawn upon, both of which involve an assessment of the impact of care-giving upon the principal informal carer. The first focuses upon economic aspects of care-giving, and how these may influence the carer's decision to accept or relinquish the responsibility. The second is concerned with the psychosocial aspects of care-giving and the impact of personal experiences upon family carers.

The long-term costs and effects upon morale are often referred to as *carer burden*. At first sight this term appears unduly negative, since many family members derive great satisfaction from looking after a loved one with dementia. Carer burden, however, does convey the subjective experience of unremitting demand that many carers report; and it indicates a need to focus on integrated measures of health, morale, quality of life and economic concerns.

People with dementia inevitably require increasing amounts of care and supervision as their condition progresses. Predominantly this is provided by family members, usually a spouse or daughter, with formal agencies providing a secondary source of assistance. Health and social care policy-makers face the challenge of determining a mix of services which both offers assistance to those who wish to look after their relative and provides formal alternatives where there are no family members available, willing or capable of providing adequate care. There are tight constraints on budgets, particularly in northern Europe, where the emphasis has been on reducing reliance on long-term residential care and increasing the length of time that people are cared for in the community. Here, the costs of informal care, both to carers and to society more generally, can be substantial and need to be taken into account. In addition, understanding carer motivations for caring may also help to develop services that are most beneficial.

Walker has estimated that across the needy elderly population in Europe two-thirds of care is provided by family members, 13% by the public sector, 11% by the private sector and 3% by voluntary agencies.[1] Informal care-giving can have great financial, psychological and health consequences. Care-givers can, for example, incur financial costs through the loss of earnings from any employment that they may have had to give up, or because of out-of-pocket payments for goods and services. They can suffer a deterioration in their own health as a result of the mental and physical strains of caring and may become isolated from their social network of family and friends as the disease progresses and care-giving becomes a full time occupation.

This has led many authors to believe that a more accurate measurement of care-giving time would lead to a better estimation of the burden of informal care, but in broader terms this is extremely difficult to define. In a recent survey of more than 400 informal carers in the UK, Sweden and Italy, estimates of time spent caring varied greatly, and 51.3% in Sweden, 4.2% in Italy and 14% in the UK were unable to quantify their care-giving time at all. Among those who were able to provide an estimate of caring time, these ranged from 7 to 168 hours per week.[2]

Risk factors for carers

Evidence of high levels of distress and depression among carers of people with dementia has come from studies of service users and, more recently, from community surveys.[3-5] The gender of the carer and their relationship to the person with dementia is associated with self-reported levels of stress. Women are more affected than men, with wives and daughters reporting the highest levels of distress and burden.[6,7] Around 40% of carers are elderly spouses, who may themselves be frail and find it difficult to manage the physical activities of caring, such as lifting, washing and dressing;[8] care-giving wives are particularly vulnerable to low morale.[9-12]

The strength of the relationship prior to the onset of AD between carers and those for whom they are caring also has an effect on willingness to care and on outcome.[13-15] Gilhooly followed spouses of people with AD over a two-year period and, although their health remained quite stable over time, marital relationships changed as the disease progressed, with feelings of tenderness, pity and estrangement replacing feelings of love. A poor pre-morbid relationship, with little emotional attachment between carer and recipient, is unlikely to motivate the carer to continue as the condition worsens and care-giving becomes more demanding.[16]

People with dementia who do not have a co-resident carer are particularly vulnerable. Carers may be unwilling to live with their relative, particularly if this means geographical and career upheaval or if they have other dependants.[17] There is also evidence to suggest that people in higher social class groups are less likely to live with the person than those in the lower classes.[18]

Access to a social network of family and friends to provide secondary assistance and emotional support has been demonstrated to be important in preventing a breakdown in care. As the illness progresses and the behaviour of the patient becomes increasingly abnormal, carers tend to have an increased reliance on family networks and reduce their contact with friends and the wider community.[19] In particular, people with dementia who move to a different area at retirement have been found to be more vulnerable, as they are isolated from other family members, have less developed social networks and have less knowledge of local services. A study comparing carers in Liverpool and rural Wales found that individuals with more years of formal education were less likely to be involved in close family networks, instead relying on wider community networks or very restrictive private networks.[20]

Little is known about the vulnerability of ethnic and religious minority groups to the breakdown of care, but the lack of information or services that comply with religious and cultural traditions and a perception that these groups 'take care of their own' may lead to more breakdowns in care as these populations age.[18]

Carers' coping styles may be useful in identifying those most in need of help. It has been shown that those who attempt to cope by emotional means, such as denial and avoidance strategies, are more likely to have a higher level of burden than those who use more pragmatic coping approaches, such as requesting information and joining carer support groups. Financial constraints may also increase the likelihood of a breakdown in care, due to the inability to purchase goods and services to mitigate caring tasks. Levels of education and professional status may also have an impact on the carers' ability to acquire information and their access to support groups and services.

Access to respite services can reduce levels of stress and prevent the breakdown of the care-giving relationships. A controlled study in Sweden found that after patients started to attend day care regularly, carers' ability to manage the task of caring improved. One year after starting day care, 24% of the people with dementia had moved into residential or nursing homes, compared to 44% of a control group who did not attend day care.[21]

Another aspect of risk to informal carers is associated with the stage the disease has reached and the level of deterioration in social behaviour. Carers looking after a person with manifest behaviour problems, such as wandering, violent episodes or inappropriate sexual behaviour, are more likely to report feelings of burden.[22] Such changes are more distressing to carers than more cognitive elements. Care-givers of those in the stage of mild dementia have reported higher degrees of burden than care-givers of those in more advanced stages, according to Grafstrom.[6] This may be due to the need for more supervision of people who are still physically active and at risk of accidents and getting lost. The carer will have had less time to come to terms with changes in the long-standing relationship than with cases of severe dementia. Grafstrom also found that care-givers in this group reported more episodes of patient abuse. In a two-year follow-up, carers who felt they managed to cope with the caring role were more likely to report decreased burden, in part due, it seems, to the progression of the illness, which in the later stages may allow care-givers more time to pursue social activities. Adaptation to and acceptance of the care-giving role had also grown.[23]

The economic dimensions

National contexts and traditions of care-giving

The type and source of support for people with dementia and their carers is determined by a range of social, cultural and political factors. The first source of help usually comes from within the immediate social network, with the spouse taking precedence.[24] Family circumstances, such as the location of children and their ability to help, play a major part in the constellation of support, together with local and national statutory care provision. In this section of the chapter, consideration is given to the circumstances of carers and the influences upon care provision as revealed in three pan-European studies.

Jani-LeBris, in a report for the European Foundation for the Improvement of Living and Working Conditions, examined the characteristics,

experiences and needs of carers of older people in 11 member states of
the EU. The analysis was concerned with support given by families to
people aged 75 and over, and not confined to those with dementia.
Throughout Europe, the family is seen as the foremost source of help to
older people, irrespective of social and socio-political structures. As Jani-
LeBris suggests:[25]

> *Virtually all social policies count on, or entirely depend on, the family –*
> *yet few member states have taken any practical steps to provide that pillar*
> *with any real support.*

The findings of the EUROCARE study on carers' experiences of formal
services tend to bear this out.[26]

In spite of a considerable lack of information on the characteristics and
needs of carers in most European countries, Jani-LeBris identified some
common patterns, including the following:

- caring for older relatives is overwhelmingly the responsibility of
  wives, daughters and daughters-in-law
- it is rare for carers to have a genuine choice about taking on the role
- even where there is little affection or attachment to the older person,
  carers are predominantly motivated by a sense of duty
- the needs of family carers for practical, material, emotional and social
  support have not been recognised
- the lack of co-ordination of social welfare services across Europe
  means that carers are generally unaware of services and provision
  is poor.

The report concludes with 29 recommendations for the improved recognition of carers throughout Europe and for the development of services
directed to their support.

A third document on family obligations in Europe has been compiled
by Millar and Warman in the UK, in collaboration with researchers in all
the other EU member states.[27] The policies of each country in relation to
the support of dependent people were analysed, and four fairly distinc-
tive groups of countries were identified.

Cash payments and benefits for informal care

One important way of assisting carers is through cash benefits which
give the ability to purchase services that they feel would be beneficial.

Across the EU, four basic models have been identified for either paying informal carers directly or providing an allowance to those requiring care which, in the case of people with dementia, may effectively be managed by the carer.[28]

Social security model

The social security model in the UK and Eire provides for direct payment to carers through the Invalid Care Allowance and the Carers Allowance, respectively. This model recognises that carers should be able to access financial support separately from the person for whom they care. However, in both countries, the levels of allowances are low and unlikely to compensate for a loss of earnings. In addition, they do not protect care-givers from future long-term poverty resulting from a loss of private savings or reduced future pension entitlements. Glendinning *et al.* also point out that this benefit confirms and formalises what are essentially private, informal arrangements; and it does not guarantee quality of care or the amount of time spent caring, and is only available to carers of working age.[28] People with dementia over the age of 65 qualify for a means-tested attendance allowance.

In Ireland, pensions and other benefits have been improved following reports in the early 1980s that 12% of pensioners were living in absolute poverty.[29] The buoyant economic climate in Ireland and very young population (with 37% under the age of 19) have meant that all pensioners now can receive free transport, telephone rentals, TV licences, and highly subsidised fuel, all of which will reduce the financial burden on those with dementia and their carers.

Social insurance model

The social insurance approach is applied in the Netherlands and Germany. The exceptional medical expenses insurance, AWBZ in the Netherlands, covers most of the costs of long-term domiciliary and residential care, although no payments are made to carers.[30] In Germany, a long-term care insurance package was introduced in 1995, which provides either entitlement to a number of service options, or a cash payment, or a combination of both. Qualification is on medical grounds, with the emphasis upon physical disability; this tends to exclude many people with dementia. Unlike the UK and Ireland, there are no direct payments to carers, with the transfer of cash between recipient and care-giver being discretionary. However, the insurance scheme protects care-givers against long-term poverty by contributing towards their retirement and sickness pensions. It also makes a holiday allowance available for four weeks respite care to provide a break for a long-standing (over 12 months) main carer.

Attendance allowance model

The attendance allowance model as found in France and Italy – *allocation compensantrice* and *indennizzo di accompagnamento* – pays cash benefits to incapacitated elderly persons. No consideration is made of the needs of the care-givers, although in Italy a companion allowance is paid in order to permit the person being cared for to remain at home. Again, as with the social insurance model, transfers of cash to carers in both countries are entirely at the discretion of the cared-for person. In Italy, this allowance is supposed to provide all the necessary financial assistance, and very few additional services are provided without charge, although some regions make an additional monthly payment to the over-65s (*assegno di cura*) to encourage care within the home.[31] In France, however, there has been a means tested entitlement since 1996 for some additional assistance in financing domiciliary care costs.[32] In Portugal, people with dementia may qualify for an incapacity pension, which includes a small allowance for both the care-giver and partner if different.[33]

Social services model

This is characterised by payments being made direct to carers, both to provide care and also to give a degree of financial independence.

In Sweden, relatives who take care of an elderly family member can receive payment from their local municipality. People of working age usually receive a salary equivalent to that of a home-help worker and, in principle, payments for part-time carers are available. There is also the possibility to take time off work to care for an elderly family member or elderly close friend, with a low compensation from the social insurance system, for up to a total of 60 days per relative per year. If the relative is a pensioner, some municipalities will provide a social care home grant instead, which can be used to pay any person that provides help, and it is not taxed. The financial costs of care, however, are reported to be typically 2–3 times greater than this allowance. There have been reports that in spite of the Swedish government's official encouragement of informal care-giving, the number of paid informal care-givers has steadily decreased between 1970 and 1991, partly as a result of the high level of female participation in the labour force.[28,34]

In Finland, home care allowances are awarded directly to informal care-givers by the 450 local municipalities. However, the rates of payment vary widely and some carers may not be paid at all.

In the Spanish autonomous region of Catalonia, there is a means tested benefit to help maintain family care for as long as possible for dependent elderly people. Families must sign a contract agreeing to provide a fixed amount of care. In the Valencia autonomous region, informal carers can apply for a means tested 'housekeeping allowance' to contribute towards the costs of care for people over the age of 75.[35]

In all countries across Europe, it is clear that the financial support available to carers, even at its best, only partially meets the full economic consequences of care-giving.

The psychosocial dimension

Irrespective of the diversity in statutory rights and traditions of care across the EU, families continue, as identified earlier, to provide most of the support for older people. For carers of those with dementia, the health, social and economic costs may be particularly high. Pan-European comparisons of the experiences of family carers provide the opportunity to assess the effects of national variations. In the next part of the chapter we consider the psychosocial difficulties and rewards of care-giving as reported by a European sample of spouses looking after their partners at home.

The data was collected in the course of semi-structured interviews with 280 spouses caring for older people diagnosed with probable dementia of the Alzheimer's type (according to NINCDS-ADRDA criteria[36]) in the past 1–3 years. Twenty interviews were conducted in one centre in each of 14 states participating in the EUROCARE study.[26]

In order to compare subjective experiences, carers were asked open-ended questions about the main difficulties in coping with their spouses' illness and the most satisfying aspects of caring for them. These are described below.

Difficulties of care-giving

Most subjective difficulties arose from the experience of loss, the feeling that the person with dementia was slipping away, losing memories, communication and personality. Sometimes the changes were so profound that the carer would describe their partner as *no longer there* or as having *become a different person*. Passive behaviours (including apathy, withdrawal, immobility and loss of communication) formed one distinct group of responses in which the partner was felt to be out of reach. Active or excessive behaviours (including aggression, restlessness, aimlessness, sleep disturbances, mood swings and anti-social behaviour) which required supervision formed the second group. Both patterns could be present in an individual:

The worst thing is that he sleeps all the livelong day, in that corner over there, his mouth hanging open. Sometimes I could throttle him. He is contrary. Recently he resists washing. Sometimes he is aggressive. (Netherlands)

He can be aggressive. We are just sitting talking and then his mood will suddenly change for no reason. He leaves the house and gets lost. I have to lock all the doors. (UK)

The most commonly expressed difficulties reflected loss of companionship through diminished quality of communication; loss of reciprocity, as carers experienced their partners' growing dependency; and deterioration in their partners' social behaviour. In common with studies reviewed by Donaldson *et al.*, non-cognitive features, and especially behavioural disturbances, were mentioned by the majority of those who were experiencing difficulties in coping.[22] Deficits in behaviour (such as apathy, lack of conversation and immobility) were more often reported as stressful than excesses (e.g. aggression and restlessness), a finding also reported by Greene *et al.* and LoGiudice *et al.*[37,38] In spite of their difficulties, the range of positive responses given by the present sample helps to explain the commitment of most spouses to keeping their partners at home for as long as possible.

Communication is so fundamental to personal relationships that more carers were distressed by the loss of understanding and conversation than by having to take on responsibility for their partners' basic activities of daily living. Sixty-eight (24%) mentioned loss of communication as the most difficult aspect of the dementia to cope with. In severe cases, this signified the loss of the person in all but the physical sense or the impossibility of communicating their basic needs:

She is not able to tell me if she has pain or discomfort, if she is hungry or thirsty. (Finland)

His physical presence is the only thing that is left. He can't express his needs and his feelings any more. (Luxembourg)

Although communication problems may be a function of memory loss, 47 carers (17%) reported forgetfulness as a distinct difficulty. Constant repetition of questions and mislaying items caused distress both to the person with dementia and the carer. In addition, confusion of past and present relationships was particularly problematic for 31 carers (11%):

He keeps harping on about the same things. Always asking the same questions. Right now he talks about the old days, he wants to go 'home', enquires about his brothers who have been dead a long time. I wrote that for him in a letter but he wearily says he doesn't understand. He knows nothing any more. (Netherlands)

There were no differences in carers' reports across the 14 countries: each sample described the same range of difficulties with similar frequency.

Positive aspects of care-giving

Taking care of a spouse with dementia demands tolerance, vigilance and physical effort at a time of life when many people might expect to relax and pursue their own interests. The progressive nature of the illness requires increasing levels of care and, despite their best efforts, the partner continues to deteriorate. This may be compounded by their partner's inability to appreciate their efforts. Fifty carers (18%) said they gained no satisfaction at all from looking after their partners.

But on the whole, positive feelings about care-giving were often associated with reciprocity for their partners' past care and affection for them; the desire for continued companionship; 'job satisfaction'; a perceived unique ability to look after their partner; and the fulfilment of a sense of duty.

Reciprocity and mutual affection

Making a return for care and affection given in the past played a major part in the motivations of 33 spouses (12%). They regarded it as an integral part of marriage and expressed no resentment of personal costs or burden. The 45 carers (16%) who felt that their efforts were appreciated by their partners were positive about their role and wished to keep their partners at home:

I can now return all the help, care and support she has given me all my life. (Luxembourg)

We had a good life together. She took care of me and I want to take care of her. Even today she smiles when she sees a photo of us. (Belgium)

We have been together for 56 years. We shared our joy, now we share our grief. Our marriage was a good one; every day I am still happy that we are together. (Netherlands)

Companionship

Being able to stay together was the most rewarding aspect for a further 42 carers (15%). When the person with dementia was cheerful or affectionate, carers reported that this reinforced their efforts. Sharing a joke or a pleasant activity, even for brief periods, was also described as helping to maintain companionship:

Sometimes, if he's in a good mood, I play him tapes and we have a sing-along together. (UK)

There's a lot of things we can laugh about together. For example, I asked her what she had eaten one day at the clinic. She couldn't remember, which she found awful. She only wanted to eat carrots from then on, so that she would always know the answer! (Netherlands)

Job satisfaction

Some carers were able to approach their new role in a practical way, gaining satisfaction from making their spouse as comfortable as possible. Both husbands and wives reported having had to acquire new skills and being pleased with their achievements. Forty (16%) found satisfaction simply in 'doing their best' for their partner:

I have the impression that she has the feeling of complete security when I am present. (Denmark)

Sense of duty

Although 39 people (14%) said they were fulfilling an obligation of marriage, this did not necessarily preclude a sense of satisfaction from caring. The traditional commitment to support one's partner 'in sickness and in health' becomes particularly important in old age. Keeping this vow could be a source of satisfaction in the absence of more intrinsic rewards:

I know I'm doing as much as I can. It's my responsibility. When you're married it's what you agree to, 'for better and for worse'. (UK)

If you have promised to take care of somebody, you should do it. I am keeping my promise to his mother to take care of him all his life. (Belgium)

It's a moral duty for me to give assistance because he is my husband. (Italy)

Qualitative data on the difficulties and rewards of care-giving, such as those presented here, may help to develop support strategies for this vulnerable group and also help to identify those carers who are reaching the limits of their ability to cope.[14]

Motivations for caring

Many individuals seem to provide care even when the burdens would seem to outweigh the benefits. This was the subject of another European study, led by the London School of Economics (LSE), where three non-random uncontrolled samples of primary informal carers were interviewed in Italy ($N = 212$), Sweden ($N = 78$) and the United Kingdom ($N = 100$).[2] The carers lived both in rural and in urban communities and at least 60% were married to the individuals with dementia. In both Sweden and the UK, care-giving was predominantly the responsibility of the spouse, whereas in the Italian sample, sons and daughters predominated (*see* Figure 4.1).

In all countries the vast majority of care-givers lived with the person for whom they were caring (*see* Figure 4.2).

The majority of carers expressed a desire to continue to provide care personally within the patients' familiar environment (81%, 71% and 77.5% in the UK, Sweden and Italy, respectively), and very few (5%, 6.4% and 4.2%) wished to give up all responsibility for caring.

This is consistent with results from elsewhere and it has been suggested that some care-givers may provide 'pathological caring', effectively being unable to leave the person for whom they care, even when formal services are provided; they also have difficulties in approaching outside agencies for help.[39] Another possibility, not often acknowledged, is that care-givers may have weak emotional ties but instead have

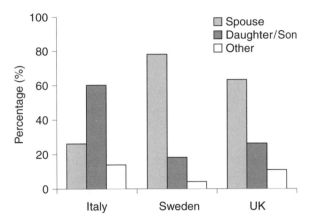

Figure 4.1: Relationship between care-givers and people with AD.

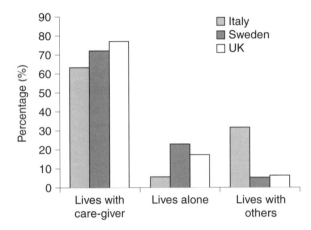

Figure 4.2: Living arrangements of people with AD.

pecuniary motivations. Alternatively, they may not be aware of, or have access to, support from the formal sector.

Although the positive feelings most widely reported by carers are likely to be psychosocial in nature, there is some evidence that care-givers are motivated by financial factors. It has been suggested that the greater participation of women in care-giving relates to the relative opportunity costs of incomes foregone by different members of a house-hold.[40] Women in many countries have fewer opportunities than men to pursue careers, due to social and cultural restrictions. This has led to a disparity in incomes; and households make decisions based on the relative opportunity costs of lost income, resulting in women usually becoming responsible for the care-giving. Orbell found only limited evi-dence in the literature to support this concept, but suggests that while income is a factor, social and cultural attitudes towards the role of women in society are also important.[17] Parents expect daughters rather than sons to take on caring responsibilities if required.

The LSE study found some anecdotal evidence that carers in the UK also take into consideration the fear of having to sell the family home in order to pay for the costs of institutional care.[41] Although UK carers were reluctant to express their views on what is, in effect, an intra-generational transfer of assets for fear of appearing to be motivated by greed rather than love, in countries where there is a tradition of owner occupation coupled with a legal obligation to make a contribution towards the costs of care, informal carers do appear to take into account the legacy they wish to leave to their children or inherit themselves. It is not unusual for sufferers to be moved into the same household in order to gain access to capital from a vacant property.

More generally, carers across Europe can also be financially dependent upon the person for whom they are caring, and fearful of losing their only source of income should the person go into an institution. Carers who are unmarried are more likely to be financially dependent, especially if they have been engaged in caring for a long period of time. A study of former carers aged in their mid-fifties in the UK found they were less able to secure employment than others in the general population and that those who did tended to secure employment of a lower status than they had prior to caring. Some of the carers also admitted they relied on state benefits, such as the carers allowance, and found it more difficult to make ends meet after caring ceased. However, it is reported that younger carers' long-term employment prospects are less likely to be affected.[42]

Across Europe, carers with professional careers are less likely to need to give up paid employment to take on caring tasks. They may have more flexibility in both the hours and the location of their work, although some admitted that they had lost the opportunity for promotion. This group also has more disposable income to spend on goods and services from the formal sector.

Carer burden and co-resident care-givers – the emerging issues

Subjective burden

Although there are positive aspects to the caring role, as shown earlier in this chapter, the term *burden*, with its negative connotations, is often used to refer to the total impact of the experience of caring. Feelings of social isolation, entrapment and loss are common.[43-45] The effects of caring, and therefore the size of burden, vary according to living arrangements and the nature of the relationship. The EUROCARE study focused on co-resident spouse carers, a group that deserves particular attention for a number of reasons:

- co-resident husbands and wives devote a great deal of time to the caring role
- spouses are on average older than other informal carers and are more likely to have physical disabilities
- the spouse's caring role is heavily socially conditioned and there may be an involuntary element
- dementia can undermine the marital relationship so that reciprocity is lost and the efforts of the spouse carer not recognised by their partner
- changing family structures have reduced the availability of intergenerational family carers, placing greater demands on spouses
- material concerns, including the costs of long-term care and the threat which this poses on a personal level to the financial security of the care-giving partner, and on a public level to a country's social and healthcare budgets.

All these factors make co-resident spouses a particularly important group in which to study carer burden.

The EUROCARE study used the Stress Process Model as the conceptual base for the study.[46] The model identifies three forms of stress or strain which can influence the experience and outcome of caring for a person with dementia. *Primary stressors* relate to the tasks of care-giving and the time taken to carry them out. *Secondary role strains* refer to role and relationship conflicts, either at home or present in the wider social context. *Intra-psychic strains*, the third form, includes the carer's subjective appraisal of the caring tasks and of how well they perform them. All of these may be positive or negative. The model allows for the forms of stress to be moderated by other factors, such as social support and individual coping strategies.

EUROCARE compared the experiences of co-resident spouse carers across the EU, with particular attention to formal and informal support, service satisfaction, subjective burden and psychological well-being. In addition, it set out to investigate the correlates of burden in this group of carers and how these varied between countries.

In terms of primary stressors, the most striking finding was a highly statistically significant association of behavioural disturbance with increasing carer burden. It appeared that this is due to the contribution of behavioural deficits, such as stubbornness, unco-operativeness and apathy rather than behavioural excesses (such as aggression, restlessness or lability of mood). There was also a weaker, but still statistically significant, association with aspects of cognitive impairment (disorientation, memory problems and language loss).

Two of the measures of intra-psychic strain concerned carers' perceptions of the extra expenses incurred by their spouse's illness and their level of satisfaction with their own financial position. Sixty-one percent of the sample reported having additional expenses, but only 31% said they received extra financial help because of their spouse's illness. Sixteen percent reported themselves to be 'slightly dissatisfied' with their financial position and 10% to be 'very dissatisfied'.

The experience of caring may be influenced by the perceived reactions of neighbours, family and friends. Respondents were asked: *How do you think people react to the illness which your spouse has?* Sympathy (35%) and acceptance (31%) were the most frequent responses; however, 22% felt that people were rejecting them or avoiding contact because of the illness. Nine percent said that others showed fear, and 2% reported laughter or ridicule.

Using the GHQ-12 to measure carer psychological distress, 58% of the whole sample were designated as *probable cases* of mental disorder.[47] High levels of mental ill health were identified across all countries. Carer burden score was found to have strong associations with carers' financial dissatisfaction and perceived negative reactions from others, but not with carer mental health.[48]

It could be anticipated that informal and formal support would moderate the stress of care-giving. However, the content and delivery of formal care provided by statutory or voluntary agencies – including cleaning, personal care, home nursing, shopping and laundry – varies between and within countries. Broadly defined, though, 48% of people with dementia received such services, generally for brief periods each week.

Input of informal care provided by family and friends was assessed by calculating the number of hours received in a typical week. Fifty-two percent of the carers received no such support. For the remainder, the average number of hours of help from family members was five, and from neighbours and friends half-an-hour per week. There were no statistically significant associations between hours of formal or informal care received and carer burden score.

The most striking findings of the EUROCARE study are the consistently high ratings of carer burden and carer psychological distress across the countries of the EU. The emergence of factors that have an effect on carer burden suggests population-based opportunities for primary and secondary prevention of carer burden on an EU-wide, as well as a country-wide, basis.

Antonovsky, in contrast to the Pearlin approach, has described a *salutogenic* model, emphasising favourable health outcomes rather than illness.[49] The focus of this goes beyond the traditional question of why people develop a particular disease to ask instead, given the abundance of stressors, how people manage to stay healthy. This is particularly relevant to the study of the impact of dementia. He has suggested that individuals having a sense of coherence (SOC) possess a psychological mechanism that prevents breakdown in the face of stressful life situations. The carer finds a degree of consistency from one experience to another; and they have resources directly under their control or to which they can gain access. All this results in a greater commitment towards providing care.

The relationship between carer burden and sense of coherence was initially tested in a pilot study in Flanders, Belgium.[50] Here, the results showed that carers with a strong SOC were less likely to manifest symptoms of distress, and more likely to develop adaptive coping methods. These findings are supported by the results of a Polish and UK study, conducted in collaboration with the Belgian World Health Organisation Collaborating Centre on Health and Action and partly supported by the EACH project.[51] Further studies, using the same research questions and methodology, are now being developed in eastern Europe and Greece: the analysis will allow further transcultural comparison, with the aim of developing a common European core and support programme for carers.

Economic and social burden

From the perspective of the informal carer, there are two principal economic costs – time and out-of-pocket expenditure. Loss of income equates to net earnings foregone, less any direct benefits that carers may receive for care-giving. Unwaged care-givers will have costs in terms of inability to perform normal household activities, such as looking after children and gardening (hence the need for substitution of paid labour), as well as having to reduce or forego any voluntary activities in which they may be involved. In addition, all carers are likely to have to give up some of their leisure time, and this impacts upon their social relationships and ability to get a respite from caring.

The costs to society include lost productivity from paid work, as well as the additional costs of healthcare due to deterioration in health caused by caring. In the study conducted at the LSE,[41] carers were asked about the level of restriction that caring placed on their ability to obtain employment. The results from the UK and Sweden were similar, with 46% and 41% reporting no restrictions of their employment opportunities. By contrast, in Italy, almost 70% felt they had severe effects. This is probably due primarily to the larger number of daughter carers identified in the Italian study sample (*see* Figure 4.3).

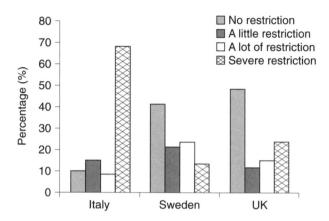

Figure 4.3:   Perception of the impact on employment opportunities in the three countries.

Direct payments or payment via patients help to compensate carers for their loss of earnings, but there are particular problems for those on low incomes. Many carers interviewed in the UK complained that they had to pay significantly more for heating, lighting, laundry and transport. In addition, they often had to make contributions towards the costs of formal services, such as day care centres, home helps or short-term residential respite care, although these may be means tested.

Younger carers, in particular, can face a future of relative poverty due to their comparative unattractiveness to employers following a lengthy period of absence from the labour market. When they reach the age of retirement they are also likely to have reduced personal pensions. Even if the state protects state pension contributions, as in the UK and Germany, no redress is currently made for any loss in contributions towards private pension funds, an increasingly common phenomenon in western Europe. Family carers in most EU countries also face the risk of losing their inheritance if a proportion of the capital value of property held by a parent must be used to contribute towards the costs of formal services if no other funds are available. They may also run down their own private savings.

In all EU countries a large number of carers are either retired or not working prior to moving to the care-giving role, but they still lose time they might otherwise have spent on leisure activities and household activities. This is difficult to measure precisely as they may be able to substitute leisure activities to fit in with caring. For instance, a carer may switch to watching videos, rather than going to the cinema if the person with AD requires passive supervision rather than active assistance.

Carers in the LSE study were asked if they felt that their activities had been restricted (*see* Figure 4.4).[2] In Italy, 11.4% reported little or no restriction on their leisure time, but 88.5% reported a lot or severe restriction. In Sweden, the result was equally split whilst in the UK 45% felt little or no restriction and 54% reported heavy or severe restriction. These differences emphasise the difficulty in estimating the subjective as well as the objective burden, particularly when this will be influenced by cultural characteristics which make comparison across countries difficult.

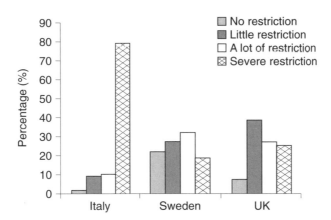

Figure 4.4:   Perception of the impact on time for leisure and social activities.

Care-givers were also asked to estimate the amount of time they typically spent caring, with wide variations in response. In Italy, 46.3% of carers reported that they were involved 24 hours per day, whereas in the Swedish and UK samples, only 3.8% and 17% of carers, respectively, reported that they were providing 24-hour care.

Living arrangements are also affected in many cases, with patients and carers often sharing the same living quarters for the first time in many years. As well as the additional stress, carers and sufferers both have to contend with a loss of space through the occupation of a once-empty bedroom. Some have argued that this space should be included in costs, as care-givers no longer have the opportunity to obtain market rents for this space.[52]

Formal support services

The provision of services to support informal carers is highly variable across Europe and within individual countries. In particular, from the perspective of carers, there is a need for all forms of respite provision, such as day care places for patients, short-term residential accommodation and sitting services, together with counselling to provide emotional support and reduce isolation.

The LSE study recorded the use of formal services by caregivers (*see* Figure 4.5).[41] The principal reasons reported for not using services were that the carer or sufferer felt the service was not appropriate, had been distressed by it, knew that the service was not available or, in some cases, was not aware of its existence. Very few carers cited cost as a reason. Equally, no correlation was discernible between self-reported ability to cope and the use of services.

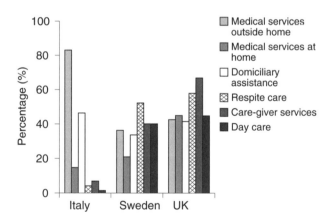

Figure 4.5:   Reported service use in the Italian, Swedish and UK samples.

A striking difference was found between Italy and the other two countries. In Italy, 83% of people with AD had had some contact with specialist medical services, much higher than in the UK and Sweden. But the use of services which might provide respite care and support was much lower, or almost non-existent. The Italian system is largely medically-oriented, and social services to assist carers are poorly developed throughout the country, with some isolated exceptions, such as in parts of Lombardy. Care-givers have traditionally been family members, and it is only in recent years that means tested financial allowances have become available. Well-informed carers who were members of an

Alzheimer's Association reported that there was little day care or other forms of respite for people with dementia. Only two regions in Italy provide places in day hospitals. A social home care package, the Assistenza domiciliare integrata, is available only in northern and central regions, providing a minimum amount of medical and social assistance to enable individuals to remain at home. Domiciliary home care is only available publicly in five local authorities.[31]

Services in Sweden are, by contrast, well-developed and publicly-funded, although carers and patients are expected to make a small financial contribution. Pensioners, who make up the majority of care-givers, are relatively affluent by European standards, receiving state pensions averaging 68% of earnings from employment. In a country of some 8 million people there are 108 day care centres for people with dementia and over 4700 places in short-term residential accommodation. A number of alternative living arrangements have been developed, including sheltered accommodation and group living. However, the population is highly concentrated in three cities, Stockholm, Gothenburg and Malmo, and geographical access to services for those living in the vast rural areas of the country is limited.[34]

In the United Kingdom, the main problem remains that of access to and quality of services, which for many depend on the care-giver's location. The mix of medical and social services is determined at the local level, and national guidelines for minimum standards of social services in particular have not been developed. Carers who have already experienced a crisis are most likely to receive help and support. Day care centres are available throughout the country and are inexpensive, with contributions usually no more than a few pounds per day. Most areas also provide some form of residential respite care. Charges for this service vary widely, some carers having to pay as much as £300 per week, whilst for others the service is free. The voluntary sector is well-developed, and organisations such as the Alzheimer's Society, Age Concern and Alzheimer's Disease Scotland – Action on Dementia – provide a wide variety of information on the condition and have formed many local care-giver support groups.

Future directions

In this chapter we have explored the motivations, difficulties and rewards reported by principal family carers across a range of European countries with different systems of support for people with dementia.

Data from three European studies of carers indicate the extent of family responsibilities expected and the commonality of experiences of care-giving across the European Union. Large gaps remain in our knowledge about the impact of dementia upon the health, morale, quality of life and economic circumstances of families across Europe, although it is evident that the location of individuals is the major determinant of the support that can be expected, both statutory and informal.

Findings from the EUROCARE study suggest the possibility that individually-based interventions (psychological, educational, social or pharmacological) focusing on behavioural deficits in the person with dementia may be of particular help in the prevention of carer burden. Interventions to enhance carers' sense of coherence may also help to reduce the subjective burden. However, findings from the LSE study suggest that access to formal support services which predominantly alleviate the physical tasks of care-giving does not have a significant impact upon the amount of care which care-givers choose to provide, or on their ability to cope with feelings of burden. Although care-givers may be aware of services, they may be reluctant to use them, preferring to provide personal care. Care-givers in all three countries expressed a strong preference to continue to care for their relatives at home, even when alternatives were available, although they did feel at times that it was difficult to cope with the care-giving experience.

Although economists present evidence of the high cost of caring and the consequent economic burden that would be transferred to the rest of society if informal care declined, traditional economic incentives, such as cash payments, targeted to care-givers to use specific services are unlikely to be effective on their own. The use of psychological interventions and training, coupled with greater access to information, are essential to a strategy to prevent or alleviate aspects of burden. Care-givers may, of course, have pecuniary motives for caring, particularly where there are concerns about the loss of a future inheritance or in circumstances where care-givers are financially dependent on their relative. Legislative measures and universal access to cash benefits, such as those announced in the British government's national strategy for carers, may help to address these concerns.[53]

In terms of community support, the EUROCARE findings suggest that perception of negative public reactions are related to carer burden, raising the potential importance of public education about dementia. Equally, the results of the LSE study indicate that awareness and availability of services and financial assistance for care-givers and people with dementia need to be improved; many care-givers were not aware of their basic rights and entitlements.

Reciprocity, duty, loyalty and affection are powerful motivations to care for a dependent family member. In the case of AD, the responsibilities of care-giving grow inexorably throughout the course of the illness. Patients' and carers' needs and preferences for support change over time, so whatever the system of welfare, flexibility and access are the key requirements.

There are strong indications that poor financial support is a source of dissatisfaction among many carers, although this does not appear to reduce people's willingness to provide care at home. There is a strong case to be made for retraining programmes for carers who wish to return to employment at the end of caring. Fear of loss of the family home or inheritance may lead some families to decline services, which is not in the best interests of the sufferer.

Focusing on psychological measures of burden alongside economic parameters can help begin to give pointers for future policy. Clearly, there is a need to identify both the costs of informal care and the factors motivating care-givers, in order to determine how best to support carers. The familiar measure of health outcomes for economists, QALYs (quality adjusted life years), cannot be applied directly to those with dementia or their care-givers and appropriate psychological measures need to be incorporated in economic studies.

Not enough is known about the effects of financial benefits in reducing carer burden. Further research is needed on the short- and long-term costs associated with care-giving, the positive and negative psychosocial aspects, and on access, demand for and use of services. Evaluations of new interventions must consider not only the impact on formal health and social care resources but also the effect upon burden and resources of family carers. This may help in developing a European perspective on the equitable allocation of resources across the member states.

References

1   Walker A (1995) Integrating the family into a mixed economy of care. In: I Allen and E Perkins (eds) *The Future of Family Care for Older People*. HMSO, London.

2   Sassi F, McDaid D, Cavallo M-C *et al.* (1999) *An empirical study of the socioeconomic burden of Alzheimer's Disease in Italy, Sweden and the United Kingdom*. In submission.

3   Clipp EC and George LK (1993) Dementia and cancer; a comparison of spouse care-givers. *Gerontologist*. 33: 534–41.

4   Huckle PL (1994) Families and dementia. *Int J Ger Psych.* **9**: 735–41.

5   Livingston G, Katona C and Manela M (1996) Depression and other psychiatric morbidity in carers of elderly people living at home. *BMJ.* **312**: 153–6.

6   Grafstrom M (1994) *The Experience of Burden in the Care of Elderly Persons with Dementia.* Karolinska Institute, Stockholm.

7   Coen RF, Swanwick GRJ, O'Boyle CA and Coakley D (1997) Behaviour disturbance and other predictors of carer burden in Alzheimer's Disease. *Int J Ger Psych.* **12**: 331–6.

8   Levin E, Sinclair I and Gorbach P (1989) *Families, Services and Confusion in Old Age.* Avebury, Aldershot.

9   Zarit SH and Whitlatch CJ (1992) Institutional placement: phases of the transition. *Gerontologist.* **32**: 665–72.

10 Morris RG, Woods RT, Davies KS *et al.* (1991) Gender differences in carers of dementia sufferers. *Br J Psychiatry.* **Suppl 1991 May** (10): 69–74.

11 O'Connor DW, Pollitt PA, Roth M *et al.* (1990) Problems reported by relatives in a community study of dementia. *Br J Psychiatry.* **156**: 835–41.

12 Collins C and Jones R (1997) Emotional distress and morbidity in dementia carers: a matched comparison of husbands and wives. *Int J Ger Psych.* **12**: 1168–73.

13 Motenko AK (1989) The frustrations, gratifications and well-being of dementia care givers. *Gerontologist.* **29**: 166–72.

14 Murray J and Livingston G (1998) A qualitative study of adjustment to caring for an older spouse with psychiatric illness. *Ageing and Society.* **18**: 659–71.

15 Sällström C (1994) *Spouses' Experiences of Living with a Partner with Alzheimer's Disease.* Department of Advanced Nursing, Geriatric and Psychiatry, University of Umeå.

16 Gilhooly M (1984) The impact of care-giving on care-givers: factors associated with the psychological well-being of people supporting a dementing relative in the community. *Br J Med Psychol.* **57**: 34–44.

17 Orbell S (1996) Informal care in a social context: a social psychological analysis of participation, impact and intervention in care of the elderly. *Psychology and Health.* **11**: 155–78.

18 Atkin K (1992) Similarities and differences between informal carers. In: J Twigg (ed) *Carer: Research and Practice.* HMSO, London.

19 Wenger GC (1994) Support networks and dementia. *Int J Ger Psych.* **9**: 181–94.

20 Wenger GC (1995) A comparison of urban and rural support networks: Liverpool and North Wales. *Ageing and Society.* **15**: 59–81.

21 Wimo A (1992) *Dementia Care Alternatives in the Sundsvall Region*. Department of Family Medicine, University of Umeå, the Research Unit of the Primary Health Care of Medelpad, Sundsvall.

22 Donaldson C, Tarrier N and Burns A (1997) The impact of the symptoms of dementia on caregivers. *Br J Psychiatry*. **170**: 62–8.

23 Grafstrom M and Winblad B (1995) Family burden in the care of the demented and non-demented elderly – a longitudinal study. *AD and Rel Disorders*. **9**: 78–86.

24 Tower RB and Kasl SV (1996) Gender, marital closeness and depressive symptoms in elderly couples. *J Gerontol*. **51B**: 115–29.

25 Jani-LeBris H (1993) *Family Care of Dependent Older People in the European Community*. European Foundation for the Improvement of Living and Working Conditions, Dublin.

26 Schneider J, Murray J, Banerjee S and Mann A (1999) EUROCARE, a cross-national study of co-resident spouse carers for people with Alzheimer's dementia: I – Factors associated with carer burden. *Int J Ger Psych*. **14**: 651–61.

27 Millar J and Warman A (1996) *Family Obligations in Europe*. Family Policy Studies Centre, London.

28 Glendinning C, Schunk M and McLaughlin E (1997) Paying for long-term domiciliary care: a comparative perspective. *Ageing and Society*. **17**: 123–140.

29 Giarchi GG (1996) *Caring for Older Europeans*. Ashgate, Aldershot.

30 Goes ES, Blom M, Van der Roer N *et al.* (1998) *Transnational Analysis of the Socio-economic Impact of Alzheimer's Disease in the European Union: the Dutch case*. Erasmus University, Rotterdam and Dutch Alzheimer Society.

31 Cavallo M-C *et al.* (1998) *Transnational Analysis of the Socio-economic Impact of Alzheimer's Disease in the European Union: the Italian case*. Bocconi University, Milan, Alzheimer Italia.

32 Poulton D (1997) *Transnational Analysis of the Socio-economic Impact of Alzheimer's Disease in the European Union: the French case*. CREDES, Paris.

33 Robusto-Leitao O and Pilao C (1998) *Transnational Analysis of the Socio-economic Impact of Alzheimer's Disease in the European Union: the Portugese case*. Alzheimer Portugal, ENSP, Lisbon.

34 Fratiglioni L, Nordberg G, Von Strauss E *et al.* (1998) *Transnational Analysis of the Socio-economic Impact of Alzheimer's Disease in the European Union: the Swedish case*. Karolinska Institute, Stockholm.

35 Pinto JL (1998) *Transnational Analysis of the Socio-economic Impact of Alzheimer's Disease in the European Union: the Spanish case*. Pompeu Fabra University, Alzheimer Espana, Fundacio ACE, Barcelona.

36 McKhann G, Drachman D, Folstein M *et al.* (1984) Clinical diagnosis of Alzheimer's Disease: report of the NINCDS-ADRDA Work Group under the auspices of Department of Health and Human Services Task Force on Alzheimer's Disease. *Neurology.* **34**: 939–44.

37 Greene JG, Smith R, Gardiner M and Timbury GC (1982) Measuring behavioural disturbance of elderly demented patients in the community and its effects on relatives; a factor analytic study. *Age and Ageing.* **11**: 121–6.

38 LoGiudice D, Waltrowicz W, McKenzie S *et al.* (1995) Prevalence of dementia among patients referred to an aged care assessment team and associated stress in their carers. *Aust J Pub Hlth.* **19**: 275–9.

39 Seymour J (1991) Pathological caring. A long-term problem that must be solved. *Ger Med.* **21**: 17.

40 Ungerson C (1983) Why do women care? In: J Finch and D Groves (eds) *A Labour of Love.* Routledge and Kegan Paul, London.

41 Sassi F, McDaid D *et al.* (1999) *Transnational Analysis of the Socio-economic Impact of Alzheimer's Disease in the European Union.* Report to the European Commission, January 1999.

42 McLaughlin E and Ritchie J (1994) Legacies of caring: the experiences and circumstances of ex-carers. *Health and Social Care.* **2**: 241–53.

43 Brodaty H and Hadzi-Pavlovic D (1990) The psychological effects on carers of living with dementia. *Aust NZ J Psychiat.* **24**: 351–61.

44 George LK and Gwyther LP (1986) Care-giver well-being: a multidimensional examination of family care-givers of demented adults. *Gerontologist.* **26**: 233–59.

45 Schultz R, Visitainer P and Williamson G (1990) Psychiatric and physical morbidity effects of care-giving. *J Gerontol.* **45**: 181–91.

46 Pearlin LI, Mullan JT, Semple SJ and Skaff MM (1990) Care-giving and the stress process: an overview of concepts and their measures. *Gerontologist.* **30**: 583–94.

47 Goldberg DP and Hillier VF (1979) A scaled version of the General Health Questionnaire. *Psychological Medicine.* **9**: 139–45.

48 Zarit SH, Reever KE and Bach-Peterson J (1980) Relatives of the impaired elderly: correlates of feelings of burden. *Gerontologist.* **20**: 649–55.

49 Antonovsky A (1979) *Health, Stress and Coping.* Jossey-Bass, San Francisco.

50 Baro F, Haepers K, Wagenfeld M and Gallagher T (1996) Sense of coherence in care-givers to demented elderly persons in Belgium. In: C Stefanis and H Hippius (eds) *Neuropsychiatry in Old Age: an update.* Hogrefe & Huber, Seattle.

51 Parnowski T, Baro F, Wagenfeld M *et al.* (1996) *Sense of coherence and burden in care-givers to demented and non-demented elderly in Poland.* Paper presented to the Annual Meeting of Alzheimer Europe, Warsaw, Poland.

52 Netten A (1993) Costing informal care. In: A Netten and J Beecham (eds) *Costing Community Care: theory and practice*. Ashgate, Aldershot.

53 Department of Health (1999) *Caring about Carers: a national strategy for carers*. Department of Health, Wetherby.

5

Services for people with dementia and their carers: an EU perspective

Sally Furnish

Introduction

This chapter provides a synthesis of different sources of information on services for people with dementia and their carers across the European Union. The primary source is the review of dementia services from a transnational perspective undertaken by Furnish and Sime for the European Transnational Alzheimer's Study, known as ETAS, in which all 15 member states were involved.[1] Additional sources are a survey of specialist dementia services undertaken within the European Alzheimer Clearing House (EACH) in 1997, also covering all member states, a set of service reports undertaken as part of a comparative investigation of dementia expert centres undertaken by INSERM and the University of Paris-Dauphine,[2] plus a literature review and direct approaches to clinicians.

The main aims of the synthesis are to provide an overview of the current position of dementia services in the EU, to make inter-country comparisons and highlight future trends where possible, and to make policy recommendations on the basis of the findings. The studies and services included are chosen to be broadly representative of the range of specialist dementia provision available throughout the EU in 1997/8. Information was included on 438 different dementia services across the spectrum of public, private and voluntary or charitable provision. Specialist services for elderly people with dementia were targeted to reflect the European Commission's funding emphasis on Alzheimer's disease (AD) and related disorders in elderly people. Some services had an additional remit towards the younger adult population with dementia. Examples of both health and social care services are included, organised under a wide variety of funding mechanisms and management arrangements.

The synthesis of information on dementia services reported here was used to develop prospectively a dementia service model. The methodology identifies the key features and components of services required by specific groups in need of treatment and/or care. Service modelling can be applied to large or small populations and is informed by epidemiological and other evidence of the needs of the group in question. In the context of this chapter, service modelling is used to identify the range of services available to this group of people and to generate hypotheses about the associations between policy, need/demand and service provision. The recommended service model is derived with related policy action points.

In keeping with one of the main aims of this volume as a whole, the person with dementia and family carers are central to this chapter, and an active attempt is made to incorporate the main features of dementia, including its progressive nature, into the service modelling investigation. In most developed countries, it has been accepted for some time that taking account of the natural history of dementia is crucial to long-term service planning.[3] An approach from health services research is adopted, whereby service responses are compared to the characteristics of need and demand in the target population, including family carers.[4]

Definition of dementia

Identifying what is meant by terms such as dementia or AD and related disorders is an important and often neglected aspect of services. People who use dementia services are not always found consistently to have evidence of a dementing illness. The definition of dementia provided by the WHO International Classification of Diseases (ICD) was adopted for the current investigation, as follows:

> *Dementia is a syndrome due to disease of the brain, usually of a chronic or progressive nature, in which there is a disturbance of multiple higher cortical functions, including memory, thinking, orientation, comprehension, calculation, learning capacity, language and judgement. Consciousness is not clouded. Impairments of cognitive function are commonly accompanied, and occasionally preceded, by deterioration in emotional control, social behaviour or motivation.*

As indicated, dementia is a multi-faceted syndrome with predominantly cognitive and neuro-psychological symptoms in the presence of global and usually progressive intellectual deterioration. The simultaneous deterioration of both physical and mental capacity poses a particular challenge for service provision. There are multiple physical, psychiatric, behavioural and social consequences of the disorder to be taken into account in planning and delivering dementia services.

European policy context

There are two main policy areas for the conditions associated with dementia in elderly people across Europe: those for older people, where the emphasis is firmly on community care, and mental health policies. Continuing care arrangements for elderly people in Europe reflect a European-wide preoccupation with the containment of health care costs.[5] Until recently, mental health services in Europe have been steadily making advances towards de-institutionalisation, but now policy is more accurately described as being concerned with achieving an appropriate balance between community and institutional provision and the related issues of public safety and human rights.[6]

The ETAS investigation was originally intended to provide a comparison between those countries with policies leading to the early identification of AD and enhanced networks of support in the community, and those which, for economic or other reasons, might favour later intervention and largely institutional models of care. Such differences between countries were found, but the *lack* of any specific recognition of dementia was much more prominently reported across the EU. This situation persisted despite considerable growth in the carer movement and a corresponding increase in the political power of carers' organisations in many member states. The question arises as to why this general lack of acknowledgement of dementia at the national policy level should occur.

It is estimated that in 1994 there were 70 million people aged 60 and over in the European Union, and the over-60s are predicted to increase to 113.5 million by the year 2025, accounting for between one-quarter and one-third of the total population. The greatest increases within the elderly population to take place in western societies in recent years have occurred in those over the age of 75.[7] This trend is likely to continue for another ten years; from 1995 to 2010, the predicted growth in the population aged over 80, for example, is 18% in Sweden, and 21% in the UK. It has been acknowledged since a spate of official reports were published in a number of European countries, starting with *The Rising Tide* (1982) in the UK, that the proportion of very elderly people in a given population is a significant factor in forecasting demand for dementia services. In line with the clearly discernible trend across Europe, the prevalence of dementia shows a steady rise with advancing age beyond 60.[8]

The policy part of the ETAS investigation found that no specific policies towards people with dementia had been formulated in any of the EU member states. This finding was only partially offset in the separate ETAS services study by the presence of broad-ranging dementia services in countries such as Sweden, where a previous history of economic capacity had combined with a political mandate to harness public funds for services to dependent elderly people, including those with dementia. Given the clarity of information on demographic trends and the epidemiological evidence, this lack of dementia-specific policies seems extraordinary.

In the ETAS review of European policies towards people with dementia, a number of general principles relating to the care of older people were derived (*see* Table 2.1), from which the policy intentions towards this group may be inferred. Maintaining people at home, supporting carers and helping people to retain maximum control over their lives are equally applicable to other groups of elderly or disabled people. It is perhaps not, therefore, surprising that the main problems with implementing policy, as identified by the case studies of most member states, included the persistently low status of people with dementia, and services which continue to be shaped by organisational and professional imperatives.

Methodology

The ETAS investigation of services which forms part of the current synthesis used the country-wide case study approach, supplemented by surveys of services and clinician interviews as necessary. The ETAS study was co-ordinated by a research team based in Wales, England and Ireland. Sources of information consulted are presented in Box 5.1.

The EACH investigation used a wide range of initial contacts throughout the EU and a snowballing technique to identify further specialist dementia services. A self-report survey of service procedures and features in relation to previously derived principles of good practice was conducted by Professor Mary Marshall of the Dementia Services Development Centre in Stirling on behalf of EACH. A separate review of the EACH raw data was performed by this author to establish the range and characteristics of dementia services. To this database were added

---

Box 5.1:   Sources of information consulted for the European Transnational Alzheimer's Study (ETAS)

- Published literature
- Organisations monitoring and evaluating services
- Formal regulatory bodies
- Policy-makers
- Professional bodies
- Carers' organisations
- Voluntary organisations
- Regional/local service commissioners and providers
- Advisory groups on service provision

---

the service reports undertaken by INSERM in Montpellier and the University of Paris-Dauphine for a comparative study of expert centres and other diverse services in six EU member states.[2] A sample of 50 people with dementia and their carers was drawn from each service. Carer well-being was measured on the Nottingham Health Profile and the Zarit burden scale; and severity of dementia was estimated by using the Mini Mental State Examination.

Further supplementary studies were designed to generate detailed service descriptions, especially in those countries and regions where information was sparse – using official documentation, published reports and direct contact. Information on the clinical presentations of people seen by services was obtained wherever possible through clinicians. Enquiries were also made about the future directions envisaged for services.

The framework of investigation is presented in Figure 5.1. It also depicts the main influences on services which were later used in the interpretation of findings towards a recommended service model. Evidence of need and demand at local, regional or national levels, and how these are estimated, was obtained. Preferences were investigated through the expectations of carers in the country, as well as popular perceptions of dementia, including those appearing in the media. Information was obtained on the following main characteristics of services:

- the range and diversity of provision
- programmes of treatment and care
- facilities and buildings for service delivery
- staff training, qualifications and professional mix
- degree of specialisation
- links between specialist services and primary care
- pathways between secondary and tertiary levels of services

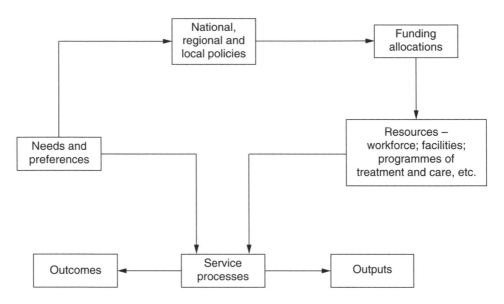

Figure 5.1: Framework of investigation.

- entry criteria, if any, for service provision at the different levels
- the responsibilities of health, social services and other agencies
- proportion of services delivered through statutory agencies.

There has been some tendency to formulate dementia service models around buildings, their size and suitability.[9] While this is undoubtedly an important aspect of dementia services, features such as the treatment or care provided and how it is delivered are equally pertinent. In the present study, research questions about facilities are therefore supplemented by items on staffing, treatment and care, and operational processes.

Nijkamp *et al.* have commented on the complexity of service delivery mechanisms for elderly people across Europe; and also they have reported that service structures for people with dementia are in constant flux, especially around the provision of long-term nursing care.[10] While the financial, legislative and administrative responsibilities for services were reported to take place at several different levels in all countries, the main policy aim detected appeared to be that of maintaining elderly people in their own homes. This was observed to have led in many countries to the development of strict criteria for entry into residential or nursing homes as a response to the escalating costs of healthcare for dependent elderly people. The importance of investigating two service processes is indicated here – the responsibilities of health, social care and other agencies in organising and delivering dementia services; and the procedures used to establish eligibility for higher levels of care.

Bleeker has suggested the use of three dimensions to describe dementia services: those delivered by a combination of disciplines; those offered primarily in residential settings or in the community; and those given by family carers, assisted by professional carers or just left to themselves.[11] These dimensions were incorporated into the present investigation, and the third was elaborated to include the type of assistance, if any, available to family carers – such as benefits, financial incentives and the range of services on offer to carers, including services provided by both professional and unqualified care workers.

Need and demand

The presence of cognitive impairment is the feature most commonly assessed in epidemiological studies of dementia. The prevalence rates for cognitive impairment across Europe have been well researched and are estimated as 4.5% of men and 6.5% of women aged over 60, rising to 32% of men and 34% of women over 90.[8] Whilst these trends are well-known, the implications are, however, generally not well formulated in strategic health planning.

Several ETAS reports, such as those from Greece and Portugal, emphasised the lack *in practice* of a systematic national approach to estimating the needs of the population of people with dementia or AD. The Irish Alzheimer's Society expressed official concerns that no formal mechanism for assessing population needs associated with dementia existed in Ireland. In Spain, regional healthcare planning involved no separate indicative prediction for dementia. Most other countries reported using methods based largely on epidemiological estimates to identify population need. Relevant socio-demographic statistics were often available but not necessarily incorporated into epidemiological estimates, although some promising attempts to integrate both sets of data around strategies for older people (not specifically those with dementia) had been made in Denmark, the Netherlands and the UK.

Extrapolation of information in relation to dementia from the national mental health dataset was the preferred approach reported for Belgium, France and Austria. When part of the information is extracted from insurance-based systems, as in France and Germany, financial bias may compromise accuracy. This also affects service provision more directly: payment loss by GPs when referring on to specialist services, for example, acts as a disincentive in countries such as Germany.

The method whereby epidemiological estimates of population need were incorporated into the development of strategic direction in dementia service provision was unclear for most member states, in keeping with the lack of specific AD policies. The present group of studies also failed to identify the use of agreed methods of interpreting estimates of need into predictions of demand for dementia services. For example, it was reported to be difficult to differentiate the needs of carers from the needs of people with dementia when operationalising epidemiological estimates of need at the local level. This may be related to the problems of understanding the impact of the condition itself; and non-family advocacy was rare for people with dementia, in contrast to some other vulnerable groups. In addition, carers had become a strong pressure group in some countries and public empathy for carers was relatively easy to achieve.

Service planning was reported to focus on the more detailed needs of local populations in countries like Sweden and Italy where there is a significant degree of devolved decision making. In the absence of a clear national strategic direction to bring together the different elements of relevant policies, a high degree of autonomy afforded to localities militated against a coherent and equitable approach. Nationally-held predictions of need and demand may be lost in the transfer to local application as decentralisation also creates more local autonomy, but fewer resources are available to fund epidemiological activity. The experience of Swedish medical professionals suggests that facilitating the development of a needs-led approach in highly localised services run by the municipalities, with insufficient input from medical and multidisciplinary health assessments, had been problematical and costly in some areas.

Information collected from those countries where the needs of people with dementia had been estimated often included comments on the difficulty of the task, particularly in the absence of a consensus around definitions of dementia and the disorders related to AD. Leading international studies have been used to provide estimates of prevalence, though incidence was rarely estimated. There is little agreement about the process of interpreting when a dementing illness constitutes a need, especially a health need, and this probably represents the wider debate about the definition of health need in those countries with policies of universal access to healthcare. Such countries expressed particular concern about affording to pay for increasing demand as a result of demographic changes and the licensing of new medications.

There are strong indications that need and service utilisation are confounded; uptake of services is often taken as a reflection of need in the population. This appeared to occur more frequently for dementia than for other groups of people with long-term mental health conditions. For example, in Greece, it was reported that predictions are mainly based on the limited numbers of people attending memory clinics. However, in most countries, people with dementia enter the formal service system relatively late in the course of the illness and there are problems of early diagnosis, as discussed in Chapter 6. As a result, the main service requirements identified from service utilisation alone are likely to be too heavily weighted towards tertiary and institutional care. Services are used to meet the most pressing current needs even if they are not originally intended for those needs. Service uptake is also affected by factors such as the accessibility of services, knowledge within the general public and the activities of gatekeeper professionals such as GPs, all of which are known to be particularly problematical in dementia services. For example, the unwillingness of GPs to refer people onward was reported to be more of a difficulty for dementia than for other long-term physical or mental health conditions among elderly people.

Reasons for the generally poor standardisation of service responses seemed to be less related to the financial systems of payment for health and social care than the process of defining priorities at national or local level. Taken together, with demographic trends towards increasing numbers of very elderly people as a proportion of the population, and a decline in the age groups traditionally acting as informal carers, detailed knowledge of the epidemiology of dementia seemed mainly to have had the effect of fuelling widespread concern about overwhelming demand on health and welfare services.

Expectations of caring

The urbanised and agrarian societies of the EU report very different concepts of family care. Families are more likely to provide full-time care for a dependent elderly relative in rural and less affluent European societies, a finding also reported from a survey of people with dementia in rural areas.[12] Apart from the difference between urban and rural areas, cultural factors appear to play surprisingly little part in expectations of caring within the EU. Indeed, there was a remarkable degree of consistency across countries in the expectation that the family should *contribute* to the care of a dependent elderly person. Depending on regional variations, this could mean either providing full-time care in the family with minimal intervention by services, or maintaining practical or emotional support to an elderly relative receiving formal care. There appeared to be a particularly strong expectation that families should be consulted, and usually involved, in decisions taken about an elderly relative's receipt of services.

In Greece and Portugal, families perceived very little alternative to caring for dependent elderly people at home. In most other countries, there was an expectation that alternatives to full-time care by families should be readily available. Objections were raised by carers' groups in those countries where families were obliged to make payments towards the elderly person's care, as in France and Germany, but families still expected to remain involved. The expectation of making a non-financial contribution was also expressed in the Scandinavian countries and the Netherlands, where the state assumes a formal responsibility for care once need has been formally determined.

This prevailing attitude of family members that they should make a non-financial contribution to the care of a dependent elderly spouse or parent has been variously described as stemming from a sense of duty, love or guilt. Whatever its origins, it is an expectation which appears to be part of European culture, finding different expression in different societies.

Low state support to carers was associated with high family responsibility. The statutory sector in Greece, for example, where no benefits are paid to informal carers, assumes a residual role, mainly aimed at filling the gaps left by families. The costs of caring for an elderly relative with dementia are perceived by carers everywhere to be high, both financially and in terms of their personal health and well-being. Yet carers have a strong sense of responsibility towards the person with dementia, and carers' groups often expressed a preference for working in partnership with services rather than relinquishing caring altogether.

Across the EU, it appears that a middle path between full-time family care and full-time institutional care is seldom available to families. Professionals working with people with dementia often have to maintain a service system in which families provide *all or nothing* care. At one extreme, an unintentional conspiracy has been described, whereby professionals legitimise the decision to institutionalise the person with dementia by encouraging the carer to give up caring *for their own good*.[13]

In most EU member states, community care policies for dependent elderly people carry the assumption that families will make a large contribution to direct care. However (and realistically), the implementation of community care policy does not rely to the same extent on families for all groups affected by it. Family ties are already broken for many of the former patients of state-run long-stay psychiatric and learning disability institutions resettled into the community, and reproviding accommodation could not be dependent on family care. There may be many other reasons for this discrepancy, including public perceptions of ageing in western societies, and the responsibilities of the state for former patients. The point remains that for elderly people, the issues surrounding the humanity of institutionalisation are seldom directly examined, and the movement towards greater use of what often amounts to institutional placement in nursing and residential homes is often justified as responding to the demands of carers. The findings of the present investigation, albeit at a preliminary stage at the European level, suggest a more balanced range of service options is expected by carers – including alternative accommodation to living at home – which promotes continuity with existing family care.

Perceptions of dementia

Until recent years, dementia was considered an inevitable part of ageing among the public and most health and social care workers. AD is now largely recognised to be a medical condition, although the syndrome of dementia is still widely confused with normal ageing, especially in the more rural and isolated regions of the EU.[12] In the ETAS study, member states with greater advancement in strategic health planning generally reported a higher level of public awareness.

Despite some signs of improvement in public knowledge about the clinical condition, there is still considerable stigma attached to AD and dementia. Perceptions of dementia in Europe are overwhelmingly negative, with only subtle cultural variations. The position has changed from one mainly of ignorance to one in which the public has a limited appreciation of the burden on families, the lack of assistance available to family carers, the mental deterioration of the person with dementia, and the most distressing mid/late-stage symptoms, such as incontinence and behaviour problems.

A mainly negative picture of dementia, and of caring for someone with dementia, is portrayed in media reports everywhere; and these represent underlying cultural constructions of what it means to have dementia.[14] On the one hand, this helps to highlight the plight of unassisted carers, many of whom are themselves elderly and frail, and may have augmented public pressure for improved support to carers. On the other hand, several professional and carers' groups have reported that negative, stereotyped images of dementia are counter-productive to the alleviation of the guilt and shame experienced by many families.

A mainly negative image of dementia also has the effect of promoting stereotypes which work against the recognition of the individuality of people with dementia. When there is also public awareness of the increasing numbers, the danger of dehumanisation and exclusion is precipitated. Dementia is feared, and sufferers may be seen as competing for a finite resource. Under these circumstances, public reactions are less likely to be influenced by humanitarian values. Dehumanisation reduces the perceived psychological complexity of the people against whom it is directed. As a result, there might, for example, be less public support for services related to the alleviation of psychological distress and the social consequences of dementia. In an attempt to counteract this possibility in the UK, maintaining quality of life for people with dementia, as an in-built and expected part of services, was central to an epidemiological report on health gain for people with dementia by Melzer *et al.*[15]

A possible connection between the oversimplifications and generalisations of public attitudes about dementia and the delivery of treatment and care was indicated by both the ETAS and EACH investigations of services in Europe. In Belgium, for example, it was reported that professional carers and policy-makers often hold the opinion that people suffering from AD cannot really be helped; and, as a result, people are not well diagnosed and do not receive appropriate treatment and care. Some groups of untrained care staff have been found to believe that people with dementia who display behaviour problems are being deliberately difficult, a belief which may be partially reversed by the provision of minimal training. The actions of professional staff may also be affected; and it has been suggested that GPs do not make all indicated secondary referrals, due to a prevailing assumption that the problems of dementia are irremediable.[16]

It is interesting to note that a wholly negative and oversimplified picture of dementia is being increasingly challenged by the responses of close relatives who have described its progression within the context of a long-standing relationship. For example, an account of Iris Murdoch by her husband, long after the onset of her AD, describes the preservation of many aspects of his wife's personality, her appreciation of humour, and her continued emotional responsiveness, including closely observed signs of her anxiety that *all was not right with her.*[17] Similar observations have been made by non-family members using an individualised, empathic approach to making contact with the person with dementia.[18,19]

The range of dementia services

Few reports of the range of dementia services exist in the international literature, although Shah and Ames identified service components typically involved in psycho-geriatric services with reference to Australia and some parts of Europe.[3] They went on to highlight additional and potentially neglected functions which might also be performed, which included:

- specialists providing liaison services in non-specialist settings such as geriatric wards and primary care
- community psychiatric nurses (CPNs) acting as case managers
- team members delivering staff training and intervention in residential and nursing homes
- educational packages for GPs.

These functions all carry the aim of bridging service boundaries, by extending the role of a key specialist.

Psycho-geriatric services are not, however, the main specialty for the delivery of secondary dementia services in many EU countries. Taking a perspective regardless of specialty, it is possible to identify a broad consensus about the functions which should be performed by dementia services across Europe. This 'ideal' range seems to be held even by those countries where very few dementia services are provided. The aspirations of countries with under-developed dementia services appear to be broadly the same as other countries. The range of service functions, and the ways in which they are typically delivered in those parts of the EU where they exist, are shown in Box 5.2.

Despite the apparent consistency in the 'ideal' range of provision across the EU, it is rarely available at the most local levels of service provision. Some of the functions are provided primarily in highly specialised tertiary or secondary services, and are not necessarily accessible to the whole population.

Some of the options listed are only demonstration projects. Long-term supported accommodation using a housing model is rarely provided for people with dementia, the main examples being the group homes in Sweden and the French cantou. The problems of incorporating demonstration projects into more mainstream and sustainable service provision should not be underestimated.

Most countries and regions are influenced by a predominant model of service delivery which exists within different compartmentalised services. The presence of segregated, vertical organisational structures has also been noted in mental health services for populations with serious mental illness. However, the relatively greater availability of community-based resources, mainly in the form of professional staff, affords more opportunity to liaise across agency boundaries. This is in contrast to the gaps in community service provision more commonly found in the field of dementia. Highly segregated organisational arrangements also mean that users are moved through the service system more often than would be clinically

Box 5.2: Range of dementia service functions identified and typical delivery mechanisms in the European Union

Services to the person with dementia

- Early identification and diagnosis (primary care services; memory clinics; specialist outpatient centres; in-patient assessment units)
- Assessment and review of needs of individuals (social care agencies)
- Financial assistance to the person with dementia (social/health insurance or social security)
- Domiciliary nursing, self-care and bathing services (mainly a non-specialist health resource; self-care may also be supplied by non-specialist social care agencies)
- Domiciliary provision of meals, house cleaning and laundry services (usually a non-specialist social care resource)
- Day or night supervision in the person's own home (a voluntary or social care service)
- Day or leisure services to promote activity, stimulation or social contact (usually provided by social care or voluntary agencies; day hospitals also exist)
- Short-stay or day admission for assessment and/or treatment (usually a specialist health resource)
- Physical and neurocognitive rehabilitation therapies (health services)
- Long-term supported accommodation provided through housing schemes
- Residential homes and specialist units attached to residential homes for long-term 24-hour care (mainly private providers – social care agencies in Denmark)
- Nursing homes and dementia nursing units attached to nursing homes or community hospitals for long-term 24-hour nursing care (mainly private providers – social care agencies in Denmark)

Services to carers

- Assessment and review of needs of individual carers (social care agencies)
- Financial assistance to the carer (social/health insurance or social security)
- Information for carers on how to access local services (voluntary and social care agencies, or individual services)
- Assistance for carers in the management of dementia (voluntary or health services)
- Short-term respite admissions or day services to provide relief for carers (voluntary, social care, health or private providers)
- Crisis intervention services to provide relief for carers (voluntary, social care, health or private providers)
- Home sitting services to provide relief for carers (voluntary and social care agencies)
- Emotional support to carers, including counselling and self-help groups (voluntary and social care agencies)

indicated for a progressive condition characterised by disorientation, where minimal disruption is desirable.

Treatment and care

There is a trend in all EU countries towards evidence-based treatment. However, studies of effectiveness are at an early stage in the field of dementia, and most research of direct relevance to clinical practice has yet to be conducted. Thus, taken together with the dearth of specific policies, the evidence that users and carers have relatively little influence produces a picture of clinical practice in the dementia field that has developed through professional lobbying and specifically funded projects. These are often time-limited, especially when not tied into comprehensive regional or national strategies. Under these circumstances, eventual reversion to large-scale institutional models of care may be more difficult to avoid for dementia than with other groups of people in need of services.

There is some evidence of newer treatments coming into practice which are resulting in a different range of service delivery. A later section of this chapter discusses new treatment and care approaches adopted primarily with family carers.

Specialist health assessment

The ETAS investigation indicated that some locations in the EU are heavily reliant upon initial specialist health assessments, followed by limited contact with healthcare services unless institutional care is indicated, at which point the main reason for contact with health staff is often to determine care eligibility – an administrative rather than a clinical function. There were few examples of community treatment models, despite the trend towards these in other severe mental illness and elderly people's services. Co-ordination of care predominantly through social care services appeared to be associated with decentralisation and opportunities for utilising public funding at the local level. Disadvantages of both extremes, exclusively healthcare or exclusively social care co-ordinating arrangements, have been highlighted.

Residential care

The EACH study identified few specific treatments as such, but some approaches to dementia care were reported. Nursing homes tended to interpret treatment as relating to medication; and regimes of care in residential homes and specialist housing appeared to range from high to low in structure and from group-based to individualised. Previous investigations have linked low structure to more individualised residential care.[20] In both the ETAS and EACH studies, particular problems were revealed in generating preventive approaches for the social consequences of cognitive impairment. 'A failure to take account of the uniqueness of a dementing illness like AD', is how one respondent expressed it. Socialisation is an important element of care for other groups of older people, and its apparent omission for those with dementia is surprising.[21] It must be stressed that this finding is indicative rather than conclusive, due to the sampling method. If the relative shortfall in socialisation programmes is confirmed, it may be linked to the public perceptions of dementia, as discussed above, or to the delivery mechanisms for treatment and care.

Stereotypes

One public misconception about dementia is that all people who suffer from it rapidly lose insight and become unaware of what is happening to them. Such a generalisation is unhelpful, because insight varies greatly between individuals and across the stages of dementia. It has been suggested that because people are naturally fearful about the loss of intellectual functioning, an over-simplified assumption of the onset of 'blissful ignorance' may make dementia more palatable.[14] Here, the priority of offering social and psychological support to sufferers may diminish. In addition, it has been proposed that the treatment of people with dementia across the EU may have been overly determined by a model which emphasises deterioration.[1] Although decline in functioning is frequent in dementia, and must, therefore, be taken into account, an over-emphasis on decline may inadvertently fuel the prevalent negative stereotypes about the condition. It may contribute to the reported sense of helplessness, even in well-staffed dementia services, about meeting social and psychological needs.[22] In the absence of evidence on effective treatment, quality of life outcomes become a major focus, especially for long-term illness.

Non-pharmacological interventions

While the potential for non-pharmacological interventions, including socialisation, to relieve stress on carers and to benefit people with dementia has been known for some time, little evidence exists regarding the way in which such interventions should be delivered.[23,24] Psychosocial approaches identified include counselling, behavioural programmes, neuro-cognitive rehabilitation, reality orientation, reminiscence and validation therapy. Psychotherapy for people with early dementia has also been reported in France, Germany, Austria and Belgium. Among the specific treatments, neuro-cognitive rehabilitation was most frequently implemented, and was identified across the majority of member states.

The rationale for neuro-cognitive rehabilitation is drawn from the experimental evidence that learning continues to be possible in early dementia.[25] After verbal encoding has been achieved, rates of forgetting may be comparable to age-matched controls.[26] The acquisition of motor, perceptual and cognitive tasks has been demonstrated;[27] and interventions aimed at optimising residual memory performance are part of this approach.[28,29] There are also promising preliminary indications that rehabilitation of memory function can form a viable component of early intervention programmes.[30] In recent years, these observations have led to the introduction into clinical practice of neuro-cognitive rehabilitation for early dementia in most member states. Neuro-cognitive rehabilitation is preceded by a detailed neuro-psychological examination, included as part of the treatment package. Because of its widespread use in the EU, a well-founded theoretical basis and its service delivery link to early intervention (a main principle of policy), neuro-cognitive rehabilitation is used here to illustrate the two main models identified for the delivery of treatment programmes.

Examples of expert models

Expert centres provide a frequently found model for early identification and neuro-cognitive rehabilitation, and have been the focus of a transnational comparative investigation.[2] These centres offer a variety of neuro-biological and neuro-psychological investigations, cognitive and physical rehabilitation, medication and combined treatments at both secondary and tertiary levels. They are sometimes developed through university teaching hospitals and are often involved in conducting research trials funded by pharmaceutical companies.[31] The specialist leadership role may be adopted by a psychiatrist, geriatrician, neurologist or neuro-psychologist, or may be shared by two or more of these professionals. Some particular examples are of interest.

The first Italian Dementia Evaluation and Rehabilitation Unit opened in 1991 in Brescia.[32] The unit houses a 40-bed in-patient facility, a 10-place day hospital, out-patient clinic and laboratory. The team represents a wide range of specialties, including, among the medical staff alone, two full-time geriatricians, neurologists and a full-time psychiatrist. Of the first 193 consecutive patients, most received a first-time diagnosis of AD or other dementia. Ninety percent were admitted from home, with 12 coming from nursing homes. By contrast, on discharge, 25 patients were institutionalised. The mean length of inpatient stay was around 35 days, and for the the day hospital, five days for diagnosis alone, two weeks for medical or behavioural treatment and one month for neuro-cognitive rehabilitation. For suitable patients without behavioural disturbance, neuro-cognitive rehabilitation, based on procedural learning, is used to rebuild practical skills. Improvements in cognitive and ADL scores have been formally recorded.[33]

A Belgian site for an expert centre study was staffed by a multidisciplinary neurological team and operated a diagnostic and treatment service via an average 2.5 month hospital admission for people with suspected dementia and behavioural/cognitive disorders. Two-thirds of the admissions came directly from GPs. Neuro-cognitive rehabilitation and behavioural programmes were combined with medical treatments. Care management, instigated at the time of admission, was gradually reduced on discharge. High risk families have been allocated a social work case manager for continuity of follow-up.

The expert centre model does not always explicitly include the option of neuro-cognitive rehabilitation. A psycho-geriatric service in the city of Munster, Germany, housed a day centre and day treatment unit and delivered home care services. The treatment unit saw approximately 33 people at any one time, with lengths of stay between two and five days. Attendance at the day centre was 20 people per day, 30% being referred from the day treatment unit and the rest from GPs and other services. A full-time psychiatrist was available, an unusual arrangement for psycho-geriatric services in Germany. Social workers ran training for professionals and non-professionals, family counselling and support groups. There were five additional day centres in the city.

These examples illustrate that alongside the treatment delivered by the expert centre itself, day or domiciliary services are frequently offered, following assessment and diagnosis, on an outreach basis, or by collaboration with social care agencies. The operations of most centres reflect a need for more active involvement beyond mere inter-agency referral to ensure the appropriate services are received after diagnosis.

Memory clinics on the expert centre model have been developed in EU countries as diverse as Greece, Austria, the UK and the Netherlands. At the beginning of the 1990s it was reported that the specialist centres for elderly people in Greece (KAPI) tended to provide medical and social care for the less disabled people, and those with greater dependency needs relied entirely on family and friends. All services for elderly dependent people were under-developed; and only 1% of elderly people were in institutional care. Specialist dementia services have begun to emerge in Greece more recently in the form of memory assessment and diagnostic clinics, but there is still a reported lack of follow-up services.

A review of the 13 Dutch memory clinics, undertaken by Verhey in 1998, shows all were founded after 1992, seven by attachment to academic centres.* The Dutch clinics offer a wide variety of treatments, delivered through a large number of disciplines in some of the units. Follow-up services after memory assessment and diagnosis are available here; and the availability of follow-up services, and how people with dementia are put in touch with such services after attendance at a diagnostic clinic, are important factors in the development of more integrative community treatment models.

The unit cost of providing the level of expertise required for a specialist secondary or tertiary diagnosis and treatment service are high, and this has raised issues of equity of access. Day admissions reduce costs but may be incompatible with the geographical area covered by most centres. Although they receive a high proportion of referrals directly from primary care sources, the rate of detection of dementia for referral on from primary care is low across the EU.[12] An alternative approach, which aims at increasing accessibility, is to provide memory clinic functions on an *outreach* basis.[34] In this alternative model, the main locus of operation of experts becomes the community, which includes out-patient facilities.[35] Preliminary findings reviewed by Moniz-Cook and Woods point to the flexibility of treatment delivered within this model, and improved follow-up rates, although there may be initial difficulties in establishing the required liaison with GPs.[36] Fidelity to treatment approaches described in the literature, albeit limited at this stage, appears to be good.

By 1998, no randomised trials of dementia community treatment programmes had been reported within the EU. The effectiveness of models of integrated care for dependent elderly people, not all but many of whom have dementia, has, however, been demonstrated by a randomised study in Italy.[37] This found reduced admissions to long-term care and less decline in cognitive functioning for subjects assigned to a service offering integrated social and medical care and adopting a case management approach. Specific community treatment services have been identified in Sweden, Spain, Denmark and the UK.

In Zamoro, Spain, a team led by a neuro-psychiatrist, has used telematic neuro-cognitive rehabilitation alongside medical care to address the problem of providing maintenance treatment in rural areas with low levels of follow-up services. In the Fundacio ACE clinic in Barcelona

---

* Verhey F (1998) *A survey of memory clinics in Holland*. Paper presented at the International Symposium on Early Interventions, Hull, 26 April 1999.

a combined medical, social care and neuro-cognitive approach is offered, staffed by a neurologist, social worker and neuro-psychologist, and consisting of an out-patient centre and therapeutic day centre. Social work assistance is available for follow-up home support services. Fifty percent of patients return home after assessment, the rest being referred to other public health services. The clinic is privately run, non-profit making and receives a public health funding contract for 500 patients per year. The average length of attendance at the day centre is three years before institutionalisation or home care management by statutory services. The clinic appears to offer families a realistic choice between these two options. The autonomous government of Catalonia has now prepared a detailed strategic health plan covering the needs of dependent elderly people, the integrated working of health and social care services and the involvement of public/private partnerships.

Other countries have expressed an interest in the future development of specialist community treatment approaches, and an EU-funded evaluation is currently taking place of the Moniz-Cook model introduced into Ireland.[38] The tendency to provide initial demonstration project funding at national and regional levels raises concern among professionals working in expert centres about the need to ring-fence special health resources when the balance of activity changes from a central unit to the community. For policy-makers, the issue has been how to provide incentives for the main professional groups to increase their work in the community – a debate which has a long history in the general mental health field. Policy-makers report that when medical professional interests are uppermost, service developments are more likely to progress along the lines of specialist units attempting to provide all clinical functions under one roof. Specialist and generic services become separated, causing some organisations to seek to manage an *inclusive* service, but with the absence of some service components, while others are well-resourced. However, professional concerns to preserve specialist health resources may be understandable, given the frequently low status of dementia services; and it is important not to oversimplify the issues surrounding the integration of dementia treatment and care services.

A further consideration is whether specialist treatments should move into more widespread use before they have been well-evaluated. The development of clinical guidelines for new medications is important in this respect, and some countries are also extending the guidelines to include psychosocial interventions. Variability of treatment approach may be high, partly because research is in its infancy, but even with greater maturity, problems in maintaining fidelity of effective interventions in routine practice have been experienced with other groups with severe mental illness.[39]

Adherence to a philosophy of care is sometimes more powerful than research evidence in shaping a service model. Among the dementia care philosophies reported in the EACH study were non-specific group or individual counselling, reality orientation, validation therapy and the promotion of activities of daily living. It has been argued that such approaches are part of the backdrop to maintaining quality of life; and a values-based philosophy of care may also help to address the problem of therapeutic nihilism among staff working with people with dementia. The extent to which dementia care is delivered in a person-centred, respectful and individualised manner will also, of course, depend on factors such as the staff involved and management practices.

Services to carers

In the ETAS study, services available to family care-givers were widely reported to be inadequate, despite the growing evidence of effectiveness of several interventions with carers.[40–42] Even psycho-educational and information approaches were neglected, and these incur minimal cost and are frequently cited as basic good practice. In the more economically deprived countries, there was reported to be no real alternative to family care, but ways of addressing the consequences for families were not formally considered, although there was knowledge in all countries of the research findings on carer burden described in Chapter 4.

Carers' organisations reported a general lack of involvement and insufficient consultation in service planning and delivery, and there were no reports of promoting the development of information systems on carers within the organisations consulted for this investigation. Again, all member states were aware of the main requirements of carers, even if the country did not provide services or financial assistance.

Respite care

The most usual service provision was respite care. Difficulties of delivering flexible care through residential and nursing home settings run on a commercial basis were identified in most reports, although some residential and nursing home services consulted for the EACH study managed to offer this in the person's own home as well. This was recorded in Finland, Belgium and the UK. In the UK, voluntary agencies, such as Crossroads, have been an active force in introducing carer relief or sitter services, the latter being an interesting example of responding to the needs of carers while also maintaining a focus on the person with dementia, since short-term removal to a residential establishment can exacerbate mental and functional symptomatology.

Respite admissions are identified as a component of residential services in Sweden, the Netherlands, Belgium, Denmark, Finland, Greece, Ireland, Spain and Austria; and day units are identified in Sweden, the Netherlands, Belgium, Denmark, Finland, Greece, Ireland and Spain. The latter are usually attached to residential or acute admissions facilities, with the exception of Sweden, where a high proportion of specialist respite was offered as part of group living, which proved to be very popular with carers. In one report from Italy, respite care was delivered within an acute health facility, although the primary reason for admission was assessment and/or treatment for suspected dementia. Respite care was not a strong feature of the French system, although some nursing homes offered respite admissions. No examples of respite care in Germany and Luxembourg were reported.

These findings give some indication of the extent of respite care for dementia in each country but should not be assumed to be conclusive because of limitations due to the sampling method and possible differences in defining respite. For example, in the German psycho-geriatric centre (described on p.106, but not surveyed in the EACH study), day centre attendance may have provided respite for carers as well as day care for people with dementia.

Diversification of services to include respite care appears to occur mainly through residential or nursing units extending their main long-term care function. In the Netherlands and Denmark, where a high proportion of residential and nursing care is still delivered through public sector organisations, such diversification had been actively encouraged by governments. Seldom had the development of respite care been led through community provision. The major problem identified was one of inflexibility – carers had to book ahead for specific lengths of stay.

Psychosocial support

While addressing the needs of carers was a stated aim of most services, the practical ways in which this occurred can be summarised as sporadic at most. Psychosocial interventions directed at family carers include counselling, psycho-education, carer training, support/social groups and cognitive therapy. Family interventions based on interactional theories have been neglected in the dementia field, despite substantial research into the changing nature of the relationship between the person with dementia and the main carer (*see* Chapter 4). This is a trend to watch for in the future. Some indicative work in the Netherlands has simultaneously provided both knowledge of the dyadic process in dementia care[43] and the development of a responsive carers' support programme delivered through home help personnel.[44]

Helplines

Carers' helpline services have increased in recent years and most countries report at least one dementia-specific national helpline, mainly run through voluntary organisations such as the National Alzheimer's Association. The EACH study identified dementia carers' helplines in Sweden, the Netherlands, Finland and Portugal.

Social support

At national levels throughout the EU, the needs of carers were generally perceived to have been badly neglected. In Sweden there have been policy statements about the needs of carers since the 1980s, and in several countries, including Ireland and the UK, Carers' Charters have been drawn up for some time but with little evidence of practical application.

There are, however, signs of improvement in the situation for carers in future. Perhaps the most promising new initiatives are taking place in Sweden, Denmark and the Netherlands, providing a mix of specific carers' services, grant-aid for carers' support initiatives, and carers' allowances, plus additional financial support, including paid leave (Sweden), payment in lieu of work, second pension schemes and tax incentives. However, the complexity of funding arrangements and eligibility criteria for continuing care make it difficult for individuals and families to claim their entitlements to benefits and services. Studies conducted in Sweden have suggested that carers prefer practical assistance from services over financial reimbursement, and that only 50% of the expected number of applications for carers' leave were actually made.[45] Implementation of national policy in the municipalities was poor, and in a recent survey of a random sample of 70 municipalities, virtually none had an explicit policy to support carers.

Voluntary sector

Voluntary services, usually run by paid workers, are often popular with carers because of their flexibility, but their non-statutory status can lead to patchy provision geographically. The UK has a long history of carer support through voluntary sector services, assisted by a complex system of time-limited development grants. Most monies have not, however, been specifically set aside for the carers of people with dementia; and the UK has been sharply criticised by carers' organisations for failure to meet carers' needs through statutory mechanisms. The interpretation of local authority responsibilities has tended to prioritise elderly people living alone over those with a carer; not a helpful position for community care policy. The situation for carers in the UK may improve when legislation attached to the Carers Strategy (1999) is fully implemented, building on the rather weak starting point of the Carers Recognition and Services Act (1995), which entitled carers to an assessment of need by request to the local authority.

Professional and staffing issues

From the ETAS study, it can be seen that the proportion of health professionals specialising in dementia varies across the EU but is related to the country's level of economic development. Medical professionals work under a number of different structures within the three main specialties of geriatrics, psycho-geriatrics/neuro-psychiatry and neurological services. There appears to be no European consensus around a preferred professional structure in respect of dementia; and many reports acknowledge that all three secondary specialties might be involved to some extent and that confusion from the practice of cross-referral does arise. There is, however, evidence from most countries that both geriatric and psycho-geriatric secondary services are moving towards an increasing focus on work in the community.

The EACH survey found that, in countries with few professional experts, psychiatrists play the predominant role; but, as other specialist services expand, these may take a lead. The main contributions made by specialist medical professionals were found to be concerned with assessment, diagnosis and an initial treatment plan, although multidisciplinary health teams more commonly delivered dementia rehabilitation services, as described in the section on treatment and care (see pp. 103–9).

The ETAS and EACH studies taken together indicate that in some countries there has been a trend of counter-specialty. This occurs at its most extreme in Finland, where the continuing care of elderly dependent people is the responsibility mainly of general practitioners, and dementia in-patient units are attached to local community hospitals run by GPs. Interestingly, the Finnish units are designed as large-scale nursing homes, often within tertiary care locations.

Despite the overall trend towards primary care-focused healthcare, there is very little training on dementia for staff. There is, however, general agreement that primary care professionals have a very important role, and that joint working between primary and secondary levels should occur. In Sweden, for example, there are community dementia nurses, whose role is to co-ordinate all services to people with dementia and their families. Currently, 21% of municipalities in Sweden have them. Co-ordination of care, as a general issue, has been identified as a neglected, though crucial, process, in the literature on community services to dependent elderly people, including those with dementia.[46]

It would be easy to see professionalism as the main cornerstone of services. However, most people with dementia in the EU are cared for either at home, by families, or in residential and nursing homes with limited, if any, specialist professional input. The evidence on residential and nursing homes suggests a rather bleak picture, and both the ETAS and EACH studies highlighted important staffing issues. The main workforce is composed of unqualified nurses, care workers or members of charitable or religious organisations. It is frequently reported that most non-professional staff, whether in domiciliary or residential services, are untrained and poorly supervised. Despite the efforts of several countries to address staff skills through national training programmes, the impact was generally greater on groups other than those who worked with people with dementia. More success in training had been achieved in Sweden, the Netherlands and Denmark, which regard this type of care as a specialist activity, and staff are more likely to be trained accordingly. These countries have retained more statutory control over their residential and nursing homes, which may be important as market forces, driving down costs in the private sector, may hit training programmes in particular.

The untrained workforce is very largely female (80–90% where estimates are available). They tend to receive low rates of pay and are generally regarded as being of low status, despite the numerous challenges of their work. Recruitment is difficult. Staffing ratios are unfavourable, yet there is known to be a considerable degree of occupational burn-out among those working with people with high levels of mental and physical dependency.

Domiciliary staff are in high demand by home-based carers and they are mainly generically trained. The inclusion of information about dementia in their training programmes is regarded as essential but difficult to achieve. More direct access to these staff by service users and carers has been facilitated recently, even in countries with a long history of statutory service provision. The provision of meals is a form of domiciliary assistance offered in lieu of or in addition to financial benefits, although the receipt of benefits and statutory meals services is often perceived as a sign of destitution and, as a result, may be avoided by some older people.

Home nursing and home care are available in all but the poorest countries, delivered through statutory or independent organisations with a variety of payment systems, most of which include co-payment by the recipient according to means. Some countries combine the functions of home nursing and home care to minimise the difficulties of determining agency responsibilities. From the ETAS and EACH studies, it appears that the availability of domiciliary services has developed in two ways: first, within the community itself, accessed either directly by the recipient or via GPs and professional care co-ordinators; and second, through diversification of the long-term care role by residential and nursing home organisations. Some countries rely almost exclusively on the activities of the voluntary sector to provide home care as in the case of France, Luxembourg and, to some extent, Germany.

In a review of six expert centres, one non-specialist Danish domiciliary service was included for preliminary inter-country comparisons – the publicly funded home care service of the city of Copenhagen, a generic service to 18 000 people. Most referrals were made by GPs, and among the sample of 50 people seen by this service were the highest cognitive disability scores of all six centres. This finding concurs with other reports that non-specialist services are often more likely to see people with moderate and severe dementia. Carer well-being scores in the generic Danish home care service were between the worst and best of the six centres. In the interests of equity, more formal recognition should be paid to the role of non-specialist domiciliary services in helping people with dementia and their carers.

The main service models identified for early identification and treatment have major implications for staff training and supervision. If neuro-cognitive rehabilitation and family interventions prove to be as promising as the current literature suggests, more extensive programmes of training and practical implementation for the main staff groups, both in specialist centres and in the community, will need to be considered. As regards care practices, an active and challenging staff development process is usually required to overcome the trend towards therapeutic nihilism so commonly experienced in services for people with dementia. Care evaluation and staff training can be combined to improve service delivery.[47] The EACH report indicates that staff attitudes generally can be affected negatively by the emphasis that most professional training places on the deficits associated with dementia. An attempt was made in the EACH study to identify services where staff training had been successful at incorporating the concept of empowering the person with dementia and their carers; little evidence was found that services considered this a priority, and yet it is probably essential to maintaining quality of life as dementia progresses.

Facilities

The proportion of elderly people with dementia in the EU who reside in some form of institutional care is steadily rising, in contrast to other people with long-term psychiatric illness, for whom large-scale reprovisioning of care away from institutional settings has taken place in most countries. This is also in contrast to the more successful application of community care policies for some other groups of frail elderly people.

Style of facilities and regimes of care are interrelated.[48] The EACH study emphasised the potential for innovation in residential and nursing home settings with regard to care practices. The principles of care used in the study had been derived over seven years from the work of the Dementia Services Development Centre in Stirling, Scotland. These included, for example, small, homely settings and staff who become very well acquainted with residents as individuals; but there seemed to be a trend towards uniformity in the larger establishments, where the regime of care was distinctly less individualised.

In the ETAS study, a concern with the regulation of quality standards was expressed in the case studies of all countries. This is not surprising when considering the dangers of abuse associated with large-scale institutional care. Both the ETAS and EACH studies indicated that as the private market for nursing and residential homes continues to expand, the efficacy of quality control mechanisms will need to be addressed.

Unlike other severe mental illness and learning disability services, there are few dementia-specific developments in sheltered housing – defined as independent living with limited on-site caretaker support. In many countries there are reported to be financial barriers to providing sufficient care hours or the level of professional care. Occasional demonstration projects of small-scale housing schemes with support staff are found in Denmark and the Netherlands, and to a more limited extent in some parts of Finland, Germany and Austria. Sheltered housing schemes for frail elderly people exist in most countries, but essentially, independent living arrangements capable of sustaining people with dementia are reportedly very difficult to achieve.

Special needs housing developments with a supported living design and providing a dedicated workforce are also rare. The main exception is in Sweden, where the Adel Reforms in the early 1990s facilitated the surprisingly widespread development of group home tenancies for people with dementia, run by the municipalities. By 1994, the Swedish National Board of Health and Welfare found evidence of a national shift, estimating that about 12 000 people with dementia lived in group homes, compared with only about 3000 in special care units for people with dementia attached to nursing homes. Swedish group homes provide a service response to the accommodation and social care needs on a scale not replicated elsewhere in the EU. They fulfilled all the principles of good quality care used for the EACH study.

In the preliminary findings of the six-country expert centre study, the Swedish group homes in Malmo were also associated with the best self-ratings of carer well-being on both measures used (Nottingham Health Profile and Zarit burden scale). Malmo has ten areas with five separate group living units of 6–9 residents each. Each group home has individual bedrooms, shared communal facilities and 24-hour staffing. In contrast, the expert centre study site most closely approximating traditional institutional care (a French nursing unit with 12 long-stay and ten intermediate-stay beds) had the worst scores of carer well-being. In both sites, more of the carers were children of residents rather than spouses, and both sites had intermediate ratings of severity of dementia among the service users.

Evaluations have demonstrated that it is often difficult to maintain people with disruptive behaviour in Swedish group homes.[49,50] Even Sweden has not managed to develop a co-operative approach between gero-psychiatric expertise and group home staff which avoids disrupting the social care model.[51] If group homes were to be adopted under public health and welfare services elsewhere, legislation of the kind introduced in Sweden would probably be required to move beyond demonstration project status.

The French model of the cantou is also an important innovation. This is predominantly a form of social care provision, although the original model included on-site health remedial professionals, but these now provide a secondary service only. In care style, the cantou is somewhere between group home and residential care, with local variations across France. There has been some drift away from the original model to include a rural design of a single small-scale domestic unit maintaining community links and usually with high levels of on-site activity. Variations now include a cluster of small-scale units on the same site under a common administrative and managerial structure. Although the number of residents in each unit can be as high as 12, a domestic participative routine is encouraged through the supervisory role of the unit manager.

An advantage of both the Swedish group homes and the French cantou is the high degree of involvement of individuals in everyday life. The cantou model seems better able to provide a 'home for life', and the Swedish group homes show particularly good adherence to independently derived good practice principles. The cantou model appears to have maintained good fidelity to the original principle of carer participation by actively involving families in unit management, including, in some cantous, awarding families voting rights in the decision-making hierarchy.

The need to maintain cost-competitiveness within the French health and welfare system has been cited as one reason for increases in the size of cantou developments. A review of European public health policy identified an assumption of greater efficiency resulting from more centralised facilities, but this lacks supporting evidence.[5] Commercial interests in the nursing home field may be at least partially responsible for a centralisation effect. The introduction of competitive market-led solutions in the UK has been criticised for a loss of equity in healthcare as well as higher transaction costs. For such a vulnerable group of people it is also relevant to take account of service costs in non-financial terms in order to conduct a realistic appraisal of future options. The hidden costs in human terms of large-scale institutional care have been identified (*see* Box 5.3), and a need for further detailed consideration of the costs and outcomes of institutional care is indicated.

Box 5.3: Hidden costs of over-reliance on institutional care

- Less flexible use of resources
- Less control and choice
- High rates of depression associated with institutional admission
- Frequently a 'path of no return'
- Limits innovation in risk management and crisis response
- Increased risk of staff burn-out
- Loss of familiar surroundings associated with increased disorientation
- Difficult to maintain family involvement in care
- Reduced contact with carer(s) who know the person well
- Difficult to maintain or establish community integration
- Increased risk of abuse
- Not a preferred option in surveys of elderly people
- Risk of public criticism

Developing a service model

Currently prevailing dementia service models are still influenced by the implicit notion of containment, whether in families or in institutions.

This is at a time when the models for other special needs groups have diversified beyond custodial practice. The situation has been at least partly maintained by the absence of a specific policy at national levels, and a corresponding lack of strategic direction. A more strategic approach to dementia services would start from indicators of need for this group which have not as yet received systematic appraisal. These include:

- the service user's perspective, including the place of older people in European society and the natural history of dementia
- the needs of families assuming the main care-giving role
- the role played by families, e.g. the expectation of continuing to make a non-financial contribution to the person's care
- the location of people with dementia, e.g. proportions of people living alone, with family, and in institutional care.

The aim of this section is to build on the earlier analyses to develop an ideal model of service structure and practice. The main features are summarised in Box 5.4, together with an implementation strategy in Box 5.5.

Box 5.4:   Main features of the recommended service model
- Improved detection of the condition
- Facilitated access to services
- Care pathways building on the natural support of individuals
- Flexible treatment and care options
- Specialist health resources
- Social care planning
- Mechanisms for integrated service delivery
- Active service co-ordination around the locations of individuals with dementia
- Practical and emotional support for carers
- Full range of services available (from assisted care at home to 24-hour nursing care)
- Supported living in domestic housing
- Improved quality control at tertiary levels

Very little evidence has as yet been collated on the user's perspective, so caution in drawing conclusions must be exercised. This does not mean, however, that the issue should be avoided; indeed, there is considerable pressure to develop user-led mental health services in many parts of the EU. It is commonly believed that most people with dementia are too impaired to provide accurate self-reports. But preliminary work

---

Box 5.5:   Implementing the recommended service model

- Develop services based on the real experience of having dementia
- Build upon existing support networks of individuals
- Bring the expertise to the person with dementia
- Sensitively inform and empower users and carers, e.g. by working in partnership with carers
- Preserve familiarity and continuity where possible for individuals
- Develop user and carer participation in service planning
- Enable the development of a community of interest

---

indicates that the sensitive use of individually-tailored listening methods can provide a valuable perspective from the person with dementia, and initial findings suggest that personal relationships, positive communication, familiarity and continuity of care are connected to emotional well-being.[52] This is understandable in view of observational reports indicating that, with the progression of the condition, the person with dementia increasingly focuses on the more immediate interactions and environment.[47] In this way, the natural history of dementia can be used explicitly to develop an appreciation of how services might respond, and the way in which personnel approach and interact with people becomes particularly salient when there are difficulties of memory and orientation.

In developing a user perspective, the expressed preferences of elderly people generally may also be relevant, although it must be remembered that they sometimes perceive a narrow range of choices due to the disadvantaged position they often occupy in society. The preferences of older people tend to be consistent with the broad aims of community care policy – the desire to remain independent and avoid institutional care.[53] Remaining at home in the face of illness or disability depends, to a large extent, upon the strength of existing community networks. The natural supports of older people are underpinned by family and social contacts providing, among other things, information, emotional support and practical help. These networks are facilitated by good housing, local facilities and shops, public transport, the activities of voluntary and other community organisations, and access to social, leisure and spiritual centres frequented by older people.

Implicit in the current public policy of most EU member states is the view that empowerment requires a two-way link between the responsibility of society for the individual and the individual's own responsibilities as a citizen. The general effects of ageing are to increase dependency on the environment in its broadest sense, whereupon the balance shifts towards greater societal or family responsibility for the individual.[54]

To maintain the independence of older people, services will need to strengthen existing support *as well as* substitute for it. This dual aim is often missed.

An example may help to illustrate this. An elderly person in the early stages of dementia starts to require more direct assistance. Family members already providing help are well placed to act as intermediaries, but to do this they require basic information about services and any other benefits. They also need information about the likely progression of the condition so that decisions can be made for the future. A lack of good information for carers has been widely reported across the EU (*see* Chapter 8). This not only represents a potential failure to access services, it may actually prevent the families of elderly people with dementia from discharging their own care-giving roles effectively.

In the current appraisal, few examples emerged of service planning based on an informed perspective on human ageing. This is in contrast to children's services, where it is often considered good practice to draw from current understanding of child development in planning services. Recommendations have been made about planning dementia services in accordance with a fuller picture of individual needs, including the progression of the condition, in the UK, Australia and Sweden.[3,14,55] The Danish Model of Care is an example of an unpublished but comprehensive attempt to identify and plan dementia services both for mild, moderate and severe presentations, and also for people with dementia and their carers separately.

Using a model derived from the 1996 UK census data, it has been estimated that 6.2% of the UK population aged 65+ have cognitive disability, including both progressive dementia and more static impairment.[56] Of these, 36% are estimated to be in nursing or residential homes, where they make up half of all residents. For those in the community, approximately 27% live alone and most of the rest live with a spouse or close family member. This method of estimating demand does not as yet incorporate the full consequences of the natural history of dementia, but it does, in practical terms, acknowledge the vital role played by the presence or absence of family care-givers, and the importance of the current locations of people with dementia. These attempts to create a more complete picture of the effects of dementia are gradually becoming more influential in service planning, but only in certain parts of the EU.

Contrary to much current practice, the needs of family carers should not be used as proxy for the needs of individuals with dementia. Families involved in caring have their own needs, which are only partly linked to the needs of the recipients of care. The care provided by relatives is usually difficult to replicate in services because of the established intimacy of the personal relationship. Loved ones will know the person's lifestyle and preferences and will tend to preserve this information as the dementia develops.

The concept of services which *wrap around* the person and their loved ones may be relevant here. Sufficient flexibility is required simultaneously to work with existing carers and appropriately substitute for them on agreed care-giving tasks. Meeting the practical and emotional needs of carers would be unquestionably central in such a service. It is this automatic acceptance of their role that carers appear to be seeking.

When family members are present, the *expression* of mental incapacity in an elderly person is largely determined by their response to the person's condition. Families have a strong influence on demand and subsequent service utilisation. Late identification of dementia is often associated with poor awareness in the family or a negligible impact on family life. A tendency not to report dementia symptoms unless they affect family life is exacerbated by the insidious onset of the condition, low expectations of services, and the finding that dementia is still, to a large extent, a condition surrounded by fear and stigma.

There is evidence that the burden of care for severely cognitively impaired elderly people falls more heavily onto informal carers than it does for physically frail elderly people with a similar degree of disability (*see* Chapter 4). Yet the availability of informal carers, most of whom are relatives, is a crucial factor in service delivery. Ely *et al.* estimated that over 55% of elderly people with cognitive disability in the UK need help at frequent and unpredictable intervals.[56] They rely on the constant availability of someone to provide such help. This level of need often occurs at fairly predictable stages in the progression of dementia; yet the majority of specialist and non-specialist services used by people with dementia lack the innovation, flexibility and co-ordination to respond effectively. Working in partnership with existing carers is again appropriate here. In practice, however, most carers remain unassisted.

The need for services usually arises in the community, although dementia also develops among older people already in touch with services, for example those who have been admitted to nursing homes for physical health problems. With regard to the former, the main issues to be addressed at this stage are those of good identification, case-finding, differential diagnosis and access to flexible options for treatment and care which maintain the involvement of existing carers. It is important to facilitate the detection of reversible conditions and to improve the recognition of dementia. Social care planning appears to be an appropriate way to assess and review needs among this group, given their heightened vulnerability. The opportunity for reassessment is required because needs can change markedly with the progression of the condition. Specialist health services are the main approach to diagnosis, cognitive rehabilitation and the treatment of challenging behaviour, and there is a consensus that specialist health services are a valuable resource which should be more accessible to non-specialist services involved in caring for people with dementia.

Most EU countries are starting from the position of a rather *ad hoc* arrangement of health and social services. Non-specialist resources have been designed with the needs of other groups in mind and, without additional preparation and training, may lack the expertise to respond to the needs of people with dementia. Detection of the condition takes place commonly in primary care and may involve non-specialist community services. There is agreement that the personnel performing these functions in primary and community services would benefit from joint working with specialists in secondary dementia services. Mechanisms to integrate the different approaches and avoid duplication are also indicated.

After condition identification, the options for follow-up services need to be flexible and well-integrated. Service co-ordination may occur at primary, secondary or tertiary levels (*see* Figure 5.2), depending on the location of the person with dementia; and the levels of co-ordination apply to all health and social services, regardless of organisational arrangements.

A degree of primary co-ordination is crucial in planning the timely input of specialist resources from secondary and tertiary levels. Secondary co-ordination is often time-limited, and may take place through expert centres or specialist community services. Currently, the preferred

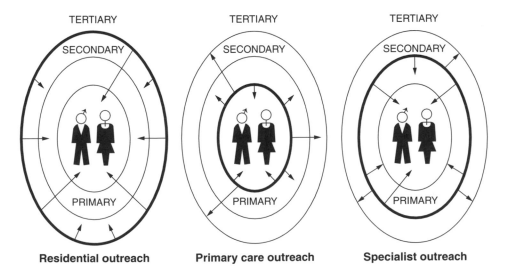

Figure 5.2: Locus of co-ordination in dementia services.

locus for dementia service co-ordination effort in the EU is secondary, with most countries expanding the role of primary co-ordination for this group. Good tertiary co-ordination will occur when residential and nursing homes actively maintain the involvement of families, and use an outreach approach, by delivering services to non-residents and forming links with other community services for the benefit of residents. A tertiary focus is required among as many as 30% of users with dementia.

The resources allocated to people with dementia receiving tertiary services are largely fixed. Nursing and residential care is financed through a variety of payment systems – individual contributions, welfare support, taxation, health or social insurance schemes – and the balance between these may alter. Nevertheless, the essential point remains that people with dementia, once admitted into tertiary care under present and foreseeable future treatment options, will not return to community living. Within the tertiary sphere, innovations are possible: dementia-specific domestic housing models have been developed; and residential and nursing homes have adopted dementia outreach to extend their boundaries into the community. However, there are also indications that more robust quality control procedures are needed to counteract the identified trend towards poor institutional practice in tertiary care.

Policy action in service provision

This final section considers what policy formulations need to be considered to ensure implementation of the service model shown in Boxes 5.4 and 5.5. These are summarised in Box 5.6.

Box 5.6:　　Main policy action points on service provision

- Strategic planning approach
- Continuity of assessment and care planning
- Public information to overcome misconceptions
- Community treatment approaches
- Joint working across primary/secondary health and social care
- New definitions, e.g. of mental incapacity

A strategic planning approach

There are very few examples of the service organisational literature being actively used for the development of future policy directions, a notable exception being the Strategic Intent and Direction approach to investment for health gain adopted in Wales.[57,58] The outcome measures used in research studies to date have emphasised the benefits to carers; for example, stress reduction, and effects on admission rates to long-term care.[59] Such measures depict service provision as a form of treatment intervention, and may have led to a tendency to undervalue any improvement in the overall quality of life of people with dementia and their carers.

For people with complex conditions associated with deteriorating mental capacity, the intended outcomes of services involve improving or maintaining health and functioning at the same time as addresing quality of life issues. These are consistent with recent policy shifts, which emphasise the contribution towards health improvement by many different agencies. In terms of service delivery, dementia is a clear example of a condition requiring the co-ordinated efforts of several agencies in service provision. When agencies are starting from the beginning with this task, there may be a need for structured approaches to service development, such as programme evaluation. Inter-sectoral action is a major component of dementia services, and incentives for collaboration across a number of service agencies in public healthcare systems are required, plus attention to accountability and funding mechanisms.

Continuity of assessment and care planning

From the work reported here, it has emerged that a number of problems arise when services fail to embody a balanced appreciation of dementia, including the medical and physical effects, psychosocial impact and the longer term consequences. The age-old debate about the nature of mental illness, and whether it should be viewed as a social disability, is being re-run for a group of people who so clearly have both sets of need – considerable psychosocial difficulties alongside physical problems. In a similar way, the well-known psychosocial implications of caring for someone with dementia have insufficiently influenced services to family care-givers and the training and management of the caring workforce.

It is possible to adopt an approach to the development of services which adheres to the fundamental principles associated with what it means to have dementia. This might lead, for example, to wider recognition that the existing support networks of people with dementia often already provide a form of protection from the deleterious effects of deteriorating mental capacity. People with dementia may come to the attention of services relatively early because of the persistence of their family, or they may be shielded from services because of the family's determination to avoid the stigma of formal identification.

There are no right and wrong courses of action where important decisions such as when to make contact with services are concerned, but families can be helped by free availability of information, and they should retain a role in decisions surrounding the person's care, even in tertiary settings. People who love and care about the person with dementia are motivated to uphold their rights and dignity, and preserve aspects of the person's lifestyle which were always important. They will also be concerned about the person's safety, a concern which needs to be addressed by regularly reviewed risk assessment, on the basis of which the intensity of the service input is modified to ensure adequate supervision of the person with dementia.

The required staffing ratios and skill mix in large-scale institutional services mean they are less likely to provide unobtrusive personal supervision. In the current analysis, user-focused services tended to be those that took account of memory problems and disorientation. Future services can build on this to wrap around the person with dementia as an individual and incorporate the existing support network.

Acknowledging the impact of the experience of dementia may also lead to the conclusion that preserving familiarity and providing continuity of care are crucial. Day support in the person's own home provided by a known care worker, or a familiar small team, would help to fulfil these criteria while maintaining the person at home for as long as possible. Such services are relatively rare. In order to provide day relief for the carer, the person with dementia usually has to be removed from their home and transported some distance. It should be noted that the service aim of providing day relief for the carer is different to that of providing day support to the person with dementia, although services might seek to do both at once. Appreciation of the user perspective in dementia is as yet incomplete, but it might point, for example, to the risk of increasing the person's confusion by providing day relief away from home. In some parts of the EU, day relief for carers is not available at all, illustrating the separate problem of acceptance that carers have needs for services in their own right.

Public information to overcome misconceptions

In considering the reasons behind the under-development of dementia services, the lack of a community of interest is a possible factor. Identifying such anywhere in the EU in relation to people with AD and related disorders proves to be a challenge in itself. In several parts of the EU, this situation compares unfavourably with the community of interest around people with learning disabilities, where several organisations, including families and individuals with learning disabilities, have presented a common set of basic demands for assistance and services, partly through the active exploration of values and service principles. The dementia service model derived from the current investigation requires both replication at the EU level and appropriate adjustment within each country, and in conducting these activities the representation of users and carers needs to be carefully arranged.

When groups of people with disabilities are formally acknowledged and recognised, the formation of a community of interest may become a natural process. The current investigation confirmed previous reports that public recognition of people with dementia in their own right is at an early stage. The Alzheimer's societies, at national and local levels, were the organisations most involved in highlighting concerns, but this was mainly on behalf of the carers of people with dementia. The role of the Alzheimer's societies tends to be one of lobbying around specific issues. Organisations representing the view that people with dementia should be afforded the same rights as other groups of people with profound disabilities or severe mental illness appear to be rare.

Development of a community of interest can be encouraged through policies focusing on the empowerment of people with profound mental disabilities and their carers, and by the use of planning methods, involving and listening to people, suited to the special needs of dementia. Public information is an essential part of the process, and techniques for the effective dissemination of information are reviewed in Chapter 8.

The difficulty of the task of rectifying public misinformation should not be underestimated, given that existing attitudes to dementia are often based on fear, misconceptions and negativity. Hopelessness is currently engendered by cultural stereotypes about, for example, an inevitable loss of human dignity. The fear surrounding dementia can be gradually addressed by providing good information on treatment and care options and a more balanced portrayal of users' lives and the coping capacity of carers.

Community treatment approaches

Services are currently organised and delivered in ways which largely maintain a contrast between family and institutional care for elderly people with dementia. Most family carers receive little or no practical assistance, a situation which persists partly because the specific difficulties of caring for someone with dementia as distinct from other forms of frailty are not fully appreciated.

At present, the EU member states make rather extensive use of institutional care for people with dementia, and future policies should take account of the disadvantages of this form of care as identified for other highly vulnerable groups. These emphasise the absence of an individual care approach which for someone with dementia can mean an irretrievable loss of interpersonal contact. It is uncommon for institutional services to deliver appropriate care irrespective of the level of severity of the person's problems, and people with more disabling conditions tend to be at greater risk of neglect or abuse. People with dementia are not institutionalised for reasons of public protection, and public opinion is usually unfavourable towards institutional care for people not considered dangerous. The question therefore arises as to whether large-scale institutionalisation represents a failure to develop alternative approaches.

Until recently, the information used to develop dementia services largely failed to recognise that there are two distinct groups of elderly people with dementia: those who have been admitted to tertiary care settings and those who continue to live in the community. Concerns about the so-called demographic time-bomb have led to an emphasis on controlling access to long-term care. Under mental health policies, a preventative approach would incorporate closer attention to those still living in the community; and meeting the needs of carers more effectively would constitute an appropriate preventive measure, as would improving standards and regulatory mechanisms in tertiary care.

What forms might the alternatives take? Two common models with other highly vulnerable groups are 'assertive outreach' and 'supported living'. The literature includes preliminary reports of proactive community dementia demonstration projects.[60] The present group of studies found few examples of assertive community dementia schemes in mainstream services. Others may have been overlooked, or such services may not be identifiable from a national perspective. The role of the dementia nurse in Sweden, for example, appears to be more aimed at service co-ordination than dementia-specific case-finding and outreach.

Supported living is a more specific concept than assisted community living. The person employs live-in paid carer(s) or receives frequent care worker visits. Domiciliary care services to people with dementia have often been designed with the needs of frail elderly people in mind and are seldom intensive enough to provide the equivalent of the care element in supported living for other groups with profound intellectual disabilities. However, the EACH study concluded that small, domestic facilities for people with dementia should be actively encouraged, and this implies the adoption of a housing model. Two mainstream examples of dementia community living, as distinct from supported living, were the cantou in France and group homes in Sweden. The Swedish model is probably closer to supported living with its innovative use of housing resources and facilities. Adherence to the original small unit design of the French cantou has drifted, although the philosophy proved to be strong in the face of market forces, and efforts have been made to maintain a domestic routine and family carer involvement.

Other important features of the care facilities for people with dementia identified by the EACH study included attention to staff training, supervisory practices and quality control. If most of the staff providing direct care are untrained in the effects of dementia, there may be a tendency for them to hold the same beliefs found in popular culture, most of which are negative and are associated with a drift towards dehumanising care. Supervisory practices are crucial because of the risk of staff burn-out and therapeutic nihilism in working with people with dementia, and respectful care practices may be sustained through appropriate regulatory procedures. Public pressure may in future help to bring about changes in care practices. People with dementia and their families frequently contribute to payment of tertiary care costs, and young payers may expect higher standards.

Joint working across health and social care

In recent years, there has been a wide range of public policy initiatives across Europe towards *health improvement* and a growing acceptance that many other services and sectors apart from health services have a vital part to play. This change of emphasis is relevant to people with dementia, who stand to benefit not only from solutions provided by services but also from broader initiatives to support their families and their communities. There is understandable pessimism that dementia-friendly environmental changes would not be seen as a priority. The environmental modifications reported in the EACH investigation were found in the relatively closed communities of segregated tertiary care facilities. But there are also examples of early interventions with people at home where environmental modifications are part of the individual treatment package.[35]

Problems with collaborative working across service agencies have been reported across the EU. Based on experience in the UK, Dickie and Iliffe point out that the most difficult collaborative working is across the boundary of primary health and social care.[61] Echoes of this problem occur in other EU countries. Most initial presentations of dementia occur in primary healthcare, and arranging community services through a social care system has the advantage of promoting more locally – and personally – responsive services. The frequent co-morbidity of dementia further points to the need for joint working.

The European studies reviewed in this chapter revealed a large discrepancy between the numbers estimated to be in need of services and those known to services. With a condition characterised by mental incapacity, self-referral is uncommon and service refusal can be high. In the interests of equity, proactive case-finding and sound diagnosis, combined with a high degree of sensitivity and flexibility in service provision, are required. The pathways into secondary specialist services need to be well-defined and accessible.

Integrated working between specialist secondary dementia services and non-specialist community services has been advocated by a number of sources. The expertise from secondary levels is invaluable in developing primary and community care skills and also in acting as a bridge across the different levels of service provision. Specialist resources are required to support good mainstream developments as well as directly serving a number of individuals. The numbers served directly will reflect the confidence and competence of non-specialist service personnel.

Failure to take account of the unique features of dementia is demonstrated by the low number of multi-agency approaches identified. Successful demonstration projects for dementia services have been reported for some time in the literature, but so far they have failed to influence wider practice significantly. It seems there are insufficient incentives for continuity of multi-agency working, and other groups take precedence for inter-agency developments. An unpublished report from the Nuffield Community Care Division in Leeds, examined the enactment of the key principles for inter-agency working envisaged by the 1989 UK White Paper, *Caring For People*. Hospital discharge was found to be the one area where these principles were relatively well-developed at the level of operational policy; it was concluded that incentives and accountability systems to encourage inter-agency co-operation were particularly poorly established.

New definitions

It must be emphasised that the recommendations for developing and implementing a service model actually require new definitions of some current concepts. What is essentially being proposed is a reappraisal of many current service solutions, and better adjustment to the problems experienced by people and their families as a result of dementia. This group is not a clearly identified body in national policy formulation and, despite the widespread nature of the condition and its effects on deteriorating mental and physical capacity, it is still frequently and inappropriately regarded as synonymous with frailty. A dependency definition is also misleading, as it under-represents those individuals who remain mobile and display challenging behaviour. The difficulties representing people with mental incapacity have also been identified in the report of the Law Commission in the UK.[62] This may be a manifestation of ageism or may simply reflect the relative invisibility of this group of vulnerable people.

The importance of harmonising the definitions and approaches to AD and related disorders in elderly people across the EU cannot be underestimated, given a projected doubling of people with dementia in Europe by the year 2050. Current solutions essentially offer only two extremes: an obligation on families to shoulder the burden of care, even when the state assumes formal responsibility; and institutional care which militates against the continued involvement of families. In this way the prevailing service models appear to be influenced by the implicit aim of containment of a feared condition. The European studies reviewed here also reveal, however, a number of promising avenues for the future which could redress the imbalance. The development of alternative, more humane dementia services requires a strategic approach, a comprehensive service model based on the experiences of users and carers, and attention to the process of implementation. There may be a specific role for the EU in co-ordinating the policy changes to guide these practice initiatives.

References

1   Warner M, Furnish SA, Lawlor B *et al.* (1998) *The European Transnational Alzheimer's Study (ETAS)*. Welsh Institute for Health and Social Care, Pontypridd.

2   Joel M-E and Colvez A (1999) *Une comparison des différentes forme de prise en charge des malades atteints de demence de type Alzheimer dans la communauté européenne: analyse de l'impact economique et de la qualité de vie des aidants.* European Commission DG V.

3   Shah A and Ames D (1994) Planning and developing psychogeriatric services. *Int Rev Psychiatry.* **6**: 15–27.

4   Ong BN (1993) *The Practice of Health Services Research.* Chapman & Hall, London.

5   Saltman R and Figueras J (1997) *European Health Care Reform: analysis of current strategies.* World Health Organisation Office for Europe.

6   Jenkins R, McCulloch A and Parker C (1996) *Nations for Mental Health: supporting governments and policy-makers.* World Health Organisation, Geneva.

7   Eurostat (1995) *Basic Statistics of the European Union.* Office for Official Publication of the European Communities, Luxembourg.

8   Hofman A, Rocca WA, Brayne C *et al.* (1991) The prevalence of dementia in Europe: a collaborative study of 1980–1990 findings. *Int J Epidem.* **20**: 736–48.

9   Judd J, Marshall M and Phippen P (1998) *Design for Dementia.* Hawker, London.

10 Nijkamp P, Pacolet J, Spinnewyn H *et al.* (1991) *Services for the Elderly in Europe: a cross-national comparative study.* Free University of Amsterdam, Leuven.

11 Bleeker JAC (1991) *Dementia Services: a continental European view.* Verpleeghuis Stetervaart, Amsterdam.

12 Alzheimer Europe (1998) *Dementia Patients in Rural Areas.* European Alzheimer Clearing House, Brussels.

13 Gilhooly MLM, Sweeting HN, Whittick JE and McKee K (1994) Family care of the dementing elderly. *Int Rev Psychiatry.* **6**: 29–40.

14 British Psychological Society (1994) *Psychological well-being for users of dementia services.* Division of Clinical Psychology Briefing Paper No. 2. British Psychological Society, Leicester.

15 Melzer D, Hopkins S, Pencheon D *et al.* (1992) *Epidemiologically based needs assessment: dementia. Report no. 5.* NHS Management Executive.

16 Iliffe S, Tai S and Haines A (1992) Are the elderly alone an at-risk group? *BMJ.* **305**: 1001–4.

17 Bayley J (1998) *Iris: a memoir of Iris Murdoch.* Duckworth, London.

18 Foley JM (1992) The experience of being demented. In: Binstock, Post and Whitehead (eds) *Dementing and Ageing: ethics, values and policy choices.* Johns Hopkins University Press, Baltimore.

19 Killick J (1994) There's so much to hear when you listen to individual voices. *J Dem Care.* **2**: 12–14.

20 Peace SM, Hall JF and Hamblin GP (1979) *The quality of life of the elderly in residential care. Report no. 1.* Survey Research Unit, Polytechnic of North London.

21 Droes RM (1997) Psychomotor group therapy for demented patients in the nursing home. In: BML Miesen and GMM Jones (eds) *Care-Giving in Dementia: research and applications Vol 2.* Routledge, London.

22 Kitwood T (1997) *Dementia Reconsidered: the person comes first.* Open University Press, Buckingham.

23 Zarit SH (1989) Do we need another 'stress and caregiving' study? *Gerontologist.* **29**: 147–8.

24 Woods RT (1992) Psychological therapies and their efficacy. *Reviews in Clinical Gerontology.* **2**: 93–105.

25 Woods RT (1996) Psychological 'therapies' in dementia. In: RT Woods (ed) *Handbook of the Clinical Psychology of Ageing.* John Wiley, Chichester.

26 Little AG, Volans PJ, Hemsley DR and Levy R (1986) The retention of new information in senile dementia. *Br J Clin Psych.* **25**: 71–2.

27 Backman L (1996) Utilising compensatory task conditions for episodic memory in Alzheimer's Disease. *Acta Neurologica Scandinavica Supplementum.* **165**: 109–13.

28 Backman L (1992) Memory training and memory improvement in Alzheimer's disease: rules and exceptions. *Acta Neurologica Scandinavica Supplementum.* **139**: 84–9.

29 Camp CJ, Foss JW, Stevens AB *et al.* (1993) Memory training in normal and demented elderly populations: the E-I-E-I-O model. *Experimental Aging Research.* **19**: 277–90.

30 Clare L, Wilson BA, Breen K and Hodges JR (1999) Errorless learning of face-name associations in early Alzheimer's disease. *Neurocase.* **5**: 37–46.

31 Wright N and Lindesay J (1995) A survey of memory clinics in the British Isles. *Int J Ger Psych.* **10**: 379–86.

32 Geroldi C, Bianchetti A and Trabucchi M (1998) Definition of outcomes in a dementia evaluation and rehabilitation unit. In: M Barbagallo, G Licata and JR Sowers (eds) *Recent Advances in Geriatrics.* New York: Plenum Press.

33 Zanetti O, Magni E, Binetti G *et al.* (1994) Is procedural memory stimulation effective in Alzheimer's Disease? *Int J Ger Psych.* **9**: 1006–7.

34 Bayer AJ, Richards V and Philips G (1990) The community memory project. *Care of the Elderly.* **2**: 236–8.

35 Moniz-Cook E, Agar S, Gibson G *et al.* (1998) A preliminary study of the effects of early intervention with people with dementia and their families in a memory clinic. *Aging and Mental Health.* **2**: 199–211.

36 Moniz-Cook E and Woods RT (1997) Editorial: the role of memory clinics and psychosocial intervention in the early stages of dementia. *Int J Ger Psych.* **12**: 1143–5.

37 Bernabei R, Landi F, Gambassi G *et al.* (1998) Randomised trial of impact of model of integrated care and case management for older people living in the community. *BMJ.* **316**: 1348–51.

38 Kenny G and Marsa F (1999) *Establishing a Memory Clinic in Primary Care in Ireland.* Paper presented at the International Symposium on Early Detection and Psychosocial Intervention in Dementia, April, University of Hull.

39   Shepherd G (1998) Models of community care. *J Mental Health.* **7**: 165–77.

40   Brodaty H, Gresham M and Luscombe G (1997) The Prince Henry Hospital dementia caregivers' training programme. *Int J Ger Psych.* **12**: 183–92.

41   Knight BG, Lutzy SM and Macofsky-Urban F (1993) A meta-analytic review of interventions for caregiver distress: recommendations for future research. *Gerontologist.* **33**: 240–8.

42   Mittleman MS, Ferris SH, Shulman E *et al.* (1996) A family intervention to delay nursing home placements of patients with Alzheimer's Disease. *JAMA.* **21**: 1725–31.

43   Vernooij-Dassen M, Wester F, auf den Kamp M and Huygen F (1998) The development of a dementia process within the family context: the case of Alice. *Soc Sci Med.* **47**: 1973–80.

44   Vernooij-Dassen M, Lamers C, Bor J *et al.* (1999) Prognostic factors of success of a support programme for caregivers of dementia patients. *Int J Ag Hum Dev.*

45   Johansson L (1998) *Caregiving and Caregivers' Support in Sweden.* Paper presented at the French Colloquium on Alzheimer's Disease, December, University of Paris Dauphine.

46   Challis D and Davies B (1986) *Case Management in Community Care: an evaluated experiment in the home care of the elderly.* Gower, Aldershot.

47   Kitwood T and Bredin C (1992) Towards a theory of dementia care: personhood and well-being. *Ageing and Society.* **12**: 269–87.

48   Lemke S and Moos RH (1986) Quality of residential settings for elderly adults. *J Gerontol.* **41**: 268–76.

49   Malmberg B and Zarit SH (1993) Group homes for people with dementia: a Swedish example. *Gerontologist.* **33**: 682–6.

50   Wimo A, Asplund K, Mattson B *et al.* (1995) Patients with dementia in group living: experiences four years after admission. *Int Psychogeriatrics.* **7**: 123–7.

51   Malmberg B (1997) Group homes: an alternative for older people with dementia. In: M Marshall (ed) *State of the Art in Dementia Care.* Centre for Policy on Ageing, London.

52   Goldsmith M (1996) *Hearing the Voice of People with Dementia: opportunities and obstacles.* Jessica Kingsley, London.

53   Nocon A and Qureshi H (1996) *Outcomes of Community Care for Users and Carers.* Open University Press, Buckingham.

54   Bond J and Coleman P (1993) Ageing into the twenty-first century. In: J Bond, P Coleman and S Peace (eds) *Ageing in Society.* Sage, London.

55   Wimo A, Winblad B and Grafstrom M (1999) The social consequences of Alzheimer's Disease. *Int J Ger Psych.*

56 Ely M, Melzer D, Brayne C and Opit L (1995) *The Cognitively Frail Elderly*. Department of Community Medicine, University of Cambridge.

57 Welsh Health Planning Forum (1989) *Strategic Intent and Direction for the NHS in Wales*. Welsh Office NHS, Cardiff.

58 Furnish SA, Bayer AJ and Rule J (1993) Specialist Considerations for Health Gain in Elderly People: evidence on organising services. *Protocol for Investment in Mental Health*. Welsh Health Planning Forum.

59 Ramsay M, Winget C and Higginson I (1995) Review: measures to determine the outcome of community services for people with dementia. *Age and Ageing*. **24**: 78–83.

60 Frazer A (1992) Memory clinics. In: T Arie (ed) *Recent Advances in Psychogeriatrics*. Churchill Livingstone, Edinburgh.

61 Dickie S and Iliffe S (1996) Working together? A research and development agenda for social services and primary care. *Br J Health Care Man*. **2**: 258–62.

62 Law Commission (1997) *Mental Incapacity and Decision-Making*. HMSO, London.

6

Clinical practice in dementia care across the EU

Brian Lawlor, Greg Swanwick and
Margaret Kelleher

Introduction

Alzheimer's disease (AD) is characterised by insidious onset and slowly progressive memory loss and can be very difficult to differentiate from normal ageing at the earliest stages. By its very nature, AD is a progressive disorder and the clinical symptoms, functional consequences and management approaches vary according to the stage of disease at the time of presentation or assessment. The stage-specific aspects of AD have been described in Chapter 1, and in Table 6.1 the clinical and management issues are also identified. In the early stages, clinical practice issues often relate to detection and diagnosis, whereas at later stages, access to appropriate services for both patient and care-giver are relatively more important.

The availability and access to new symptomatic treatments is becoming increasingly relevant at all stages of the illness, but most particularly at the early stage. Appropriate clinical practice models for AD and other dementias, of necessity, must involve close co-operation and collaboration between primary care and secondary care at all stages of the illness.

With the demographic shift and increasing proportion of elderly across Europe, it is predicted that the numbers of elderly people with dementia, and in particular AD, will double by the middle of the twenty-first century. Changes in the care-giver demographic profile, together with greater female involvement in the workforce, also suggest a decline in the number of family care-givers. Both of these changes

Table 6.1: Time-line for the development of AD

	Pre-clinical stage	Early clinical stage	Middle clinical stage	Late clinical stage
Pathology time-line	*Diffuse plaques*	*Neuritic plaques, tangles, neuronal and synaptic loss*		
	?20 years	3–5 years	3–5 years	5–8 years
Stages	**Pre-clinical stage** ? Depressive features Subjective memory complaints	**Early clinical stage** Mild memory loss for recent events Mild word finding difficulties Deterioration in higher order instrumental activities of daily living (e.g. money management)	**Middle clinical stage** More obvious memory difficulties Receptive and expressive language problems Gradual erosion of all instrumental activities of daily living, needing supervision at home Behavioural and psychiatric complications	**Late clinical stage** Continued loss of short- and long-term memory Problems with basic activities of daily living (dressing, toileting, feeding) Deterioration in mobility Death from pneumonia or other infection Behavioural and psychiatric complications
Clinical and management issues	Pre-symptomatic diagnosis Genetic risk assessment	Detection and diagnosis Disclosure of diagnosis Education, support, advance directives, symptomatic and disease-modifying treatment	Education, support, symptomatic treatment (including behavioural and psychiatric symptoms), day care, respite care	Education, support, management of symptoms, respite care and long-term care options
	Asymptomatic	**Early symptoms**	**Middle symptoms**	**Late symptoms**

occurring together will increase the seriousness of the care problem created by AD and other dementias unless there is a dramatic therapeutic breakthrough that either arrests or delays the progression of the disease.

Detection and diagnosis of dementia

Despite the growing public awareness of the problems presented by AD, it has been known for some time that primary care physicians and families frequently overlook mild dementia and that many dementia sufferers do not receive medical attention until an advanced stage.[1]

There are several possible explanations for late detection and diagnosis in primary care settings. In the earliest stages, the mild memory loss of AD can be difficult to differentiate from normal ageing and may not worry many patients or their care-givers. At this stage, memory problems are often attributed to the ageing process and ignored or minimised and may not be brought to the attention of the primary care physician. These so-called 'silent dementia' cases remain undetected and undiagnosed.[2] Even when memory loss is more obvious, the care-giver may be aware that there is a problem that warrants a visit to the GP, but the patient may be unaware of the deficits and refuse to have the problem investigated.

Lack of awareness of the illness – thought to be due to involvement of specific brain areas by the disease process, as opposed to denial of the illness – is a unique aspect of dementia and AD that further complicates the assessment, diagnosis and management. Based on the false assumption that little can be done for mildly demented patients, most health services concentrate their resources on intervening in crisis situations, providing permanent care facilities or control of behavioural complications for patients with advanced dementia.[1] Unfortunately, at such a late stage the prevalence of multiple complications is high and the prognosis is poor.[3]

Dementia and primary care across Europe: comparative evidence

There is little published information available on dementia care practice amongst primary care doctors in individual countries in Europe. A German survey found that dementia is under-diagnosed in primary

care and that memory disturbances are mainly regarded as consequences of cerebrovascular disease.[4] The same group reported that over
60% of primary care physicians would prescribe cognitive enhancers to
patients with mild or moderate memory problems, despite major doubts
as to their efficacy.[5] A Spanish study has reported that the majority of
GPs were not familiar with the initial symptoms of dementia and had
little knowledge of management options other than specialist referral.[6]
This report also suggested that they had poor knowledge of dementia
aetiologies, and 40% believed it to be curable. A survey carried out by the
Alzheimer's Disease Society in the UK indicated that in the demanding
context of primary care, GPs were unable to provide reliable diagnoses of
AD and other dementias.[7] A Scottish survey reported that the majority
of GPs felt that they had little to offer dementia patients and that early
referral was unhelpful.[8]

A recent postal survey conducted by the European Alzheimer Clearing
House (EACH) in all European countries found that the level of knowledge about dementia among primary care physicians needed to be
improved considerably, particularly in the area of differential diagnosis,
genetics and treatment. There were also gaps in the knowledge base
regarding referral to services and how to provide information, and
assessment approaches did not involve formal cognitive assessment for
the most part. However, the findings from this postal survey must be
interpreted with caution, considering the very low response rate of 8%.

Given the sparsity of knowledge, there is a clear need for more comparative information on dementia care practice across Europe. In 1997,
a European Transnational Study on Alzheimer's disease (ETAS) involving all 15 European Union countries was initiated to study policy and
practice in dementia care across Europe. One of the primary aims of
ETAS was to address this dearth of European evidence on dementia care
practice. In the ETAS study, qualitative information on the current state
of clinical practice was gathered by case study writers in each country,
using interviews of key clinical personnel and a review of the literature.[9]
A list of topic areas was provided to each case writer in order to gather
comparable information from each country. Published data on the relevant areas was also identified, where possible, and used to complete the
reports. Of necessity, much of the information obtained was impression-
istic and derived from 'expert' sources.

Five key areas pertaining to clinical practice were examined: the state
of dementia care services; the level of specialist development; methods of
detection, diagnosis and assessment of dementia in primary care and
secondary care; the practice relating to disclosure of diagnosis; and the
availability and prescribing pattern of cholinesterase inhibitors. In order
to compare dementia care, aspects of practice were classified descriptively

into broad categories of maturity, as outlined below. While there are inherent flaws in such a classification system, it allows some useful comparisons to be made across countries.

Dementia services

Dementia care practice can be defined as the model of service provision available in a particular country for patients with dementia from the time of diagnosis to death. The stages of development of dementia care practice can be classified into four broad categories, from that at a very early stage through to where there is a very high level of sophistication. These descriptive stages, rated from 1 to 4, are shown below:

- *Stage 1* – only basic dementia services available, if at all, and those that do exist are usually in general (psychiatric) facilities only.
- *Stage 2* – separate and/or specialised geriatric programmes beginning to be established, including long-term care and community-based programmes.
- *Stage 3* – full range of long-term, hospital-based and community-based geriatric programmes exist in many parts of the country.
- *Stage 4* – entire spectrum of services exist with multidisciplinary team involvement, hospital and community integration, co-operation throughout the country and equitable access to all in need.

As expected, dementia care practice is at varying stages of development across Europe (*see* Table 6.2). No country has achieved the highest level, and most countries are at the second stage only. A number of countries, including Sweden, Denmark, Netherlands, Finland and the UK, have developed dementia care across the range of community, hospital and long-term residential care. However, even here there are continuing gaps in terms of regional variation, and difficulties with liaison and co-operation between each of the different service components and providers.

Specialists in dementia care

The level of specialist care delivered to individuals with dementia and their care-givers mirrors to some extent the development of geriatrics and geriatric psychiatry across the different countries. It is important,

Table 6.2: Stage of development of services for people with dementia in the EU

Country	Stage of development
Denmark	3
Finland	3
The Netherlands	3
Sweden	3
UK	3
Germany	2–3
Ireland	2–3
Belgium	2
France	2
Italy	2
Luxembourg	2
Spain	2
Austria	1–2
Greece	1
Portugal	1

therefore, to know about this in each country when making comparisons of clinical practice across Europe.

The number and type of specialists involved in the assessment, diagnosis and treatment of dementia patients varies across Europe. The development of specialists involved in dementia care was classified according to whether there was accreditation or certification for that specialty in a particular country, and whether adequate numbers to meet the country's needs were in place. The lowest stage of development existed where there were no specialists designated, and the highest was where there were adequate numbers of specialists throughout the particular country to meet the needs of the population.

- *Stage 1* – no standardised, objectively assessed criteria exist for the designation of old age psychiatrists, geriatricians, neurologists and community nurses.
- *Stage 2* – accreditation/certification processes for the relevant specialties (geriatrics, old age psychiatry, neurology) exist and are well-accepted by the professional communities and Department of Health, but no adequate assessment has been made of the required number of such staff.
- *Stage 3* – as Stage 2, but the estimated requirement for specialist personnel in geriatrics and related specialties has been established; however, such staff are not yet in place, and gaps exist.
- *Stage 4* – as Stage 2, but the full complement of specialists required to meet the needs of the country is in place.

Using this system, a number of findings emerge (*see* Table 6.3). First, geriatrics is a recognised specialty in all but two of the 15 countries examined. Surprisingly, however, geriatric psychiatry is recognised as a specialty in only one-third of countries. Where dementia care is at an early stage of development, there tends to be little or even no specialist development. However, in certain countries, such as Sweden and Denmark, while there is no specialisation in geriatric psychiatry, there is nevertheless a highly specialised geriatric system in place, together with a relatively sophisticated level of dementia care, and geriatricians carry out the bulk of dementia assessments in secondary care. While the level of service under these circumstances is generally high, the lack of recognition of geriatric psychiatry as a specialty could result in a deficit in training skills and personnel to deal with the behavioural and psychiatric symptoms complicating dementia.

In some countries – Finland and Spain, for example – neurologists are prominent in terms of assessment of dementia in secondary care. In others, such as the UK and Ireland, geriatricians tend to see dementia cases with medical problems, old age psychiatrists see patients with behavioural and psychiatric problems, while neurologists assess early onset cases.

Table 6.3: Stage of development of specialists in dementia in the EU

Country	Stage of development
Finland	3
The Netherlands	3
UK	3
Ireland	2–3
Denmark	2
Sweden	2
Austria	1–2
Belgium	1–2
France	1–2
Germany	1–2
Italy	1–2
Luxembourg	1–2
Spain	1–2
Greece	1
Portugal	1

With regard to the use of assessment tools and instruments by secondary care specialists throughout Europe, neurologists, geriatricians and old age psychiatrists, where they exist, show familiarity with the internationally accepted screening tools and standardised criteria for dementia. The most commonly used appears to be the Folstein Mini-Mental State Examination (MMSE).

Making the diagnosis of dementia in primary care

As highlighted earlier, dementia tends to be diagnosed at a late stage in primary care settings and the level of knowledge about dementia is low among GPs. The ETAS study attempted to clarify how GPs assessed and diagnosed dementia across Europe and to identify what gaps or deficits exist in clinical practice. To allow comparison across countries, a four point rating system was used, which classified the level of sophistication used in diagnosing and detecting dementia.

- *Level 1* – the diagnosis of dementia or AD is not routinely made, cognitive screening tests are not used, and no national guidelines exist for the detection and diagnosis of dementia in primary care.
- *Level 2* – a clinical diagnosis of dementia based on symptoms is made, but only when a problem arises, use of cognitive screening tests on a routine basis is not widely accepted, no attempts are made to subtype the dementia, and either there are no guidelines for the detection and diagnosis of dementia in primary care or, if such guidelines exist, they are rarely used.
- *Level 3* – the diagnosis of dementia based on clinical symptoms and cognitive screening tests occurs in many parts of the country, AD is differentiated from vascular dementia or other treatable/arrestable causes of dementia, and practice guidelines for detection and diagnosis of dementia have been developed and are in use in parts of the country.
- *Level 4* – the diagnosis of dementia is routinely made, based on clinical symptoms and cognitive screening tests, subtyping between AD and vascular dementia occurs, and practice guidelines for primary care are widely used nationwide.

In general, the level of sophistication applied to the detection of dementia is low across Europe (*see* Table 6.4). GPs tend to diagnose it based on symptoms only, and for the most part they do not use cognitive screening tools and guidelines, or differentiate between vascular dementia and AD. GPs tend to see dementia patients late in the course of their illness

Table 6.4: Making the diagnosis of AD in primary care

Country	Level of sophistication
UK	2–3
Austria	2
Belgium	2
Denmark	2
Finland	2
France	2
Germany	2
Greece	2
The Netherlands	2
Ireland	2
Italy	2
Luxembourg	2
Spain	2
Sweden	2
Portugal	1

and usually only when they or their family have recognised a chronic problem. Four countries – Ireland, the UK, the Netherlands and Finland – have guidelines for primary care, but GPs rarely use them.

In a number of countries, notably France and the UK, there was published evidence of a low rate of use of cognitive screening tools such as the MMSE. In Sweden and Denmark, it was noted that a significant number of patients were in contact with dementia services without a formal diagnosis by a doctor.

Many countries indicated, in addition, that younger patients were referred from primary care earlier in the disease process than were older patients. Although there was no published evidence for this, in Finland, for example, GP guidelines recommend referral of patients aged under 75. Interestingly, very few countries – the UK and Germany being notable exceptions – provide dedicated services for early onset dementia cases. Even in those countries where such services exist, they occur on a sporadic basis.

Disclosing the diagnosis in primary and secondary care

As indicated in Chapter 3, there is a growing interest in the vexed question of disclosing the diagnosis of AD.[10–12] It is essential that the diagnosis be discussed frankly, while the patient remains competent. However, Vassilas and Donaldson reported on the findings from a survey of 372 GPs that showed they were more likely to inform patients of a diagnosis of cancer than one of dementia.[13] Psychological distress is the main argument for withholding information. But there is a paradox: whilst most care-givers do not want their relative to be told, they would wish to be told themselves if they were in the same situation.[12]

This issue was explored further in the ETAS study by soliciting the opinions of experts in each of the countries regarding the practice usually followed by most specialists. While the assessment and diagnostic methods used in secondary care differ very little across the EU, *how* the diagnosis is disclosed, and to *whom*, varies considerably. This is shown in Table 6.5.

Table 6.5: Disclosure of the diagnosis of AD in secondary care

Country	No disclosure	To family only	Always to family, sometimes to patient	Always to both patient and family
Austria		✓		
Belgium			✓	
Denmark				✓
Finland				✓
France			✓	
Germany				✓
Greece		✓		
Holland			✓	
Ireland			✓	
Italy			✓	
Luxembourg			✓	
Portugal		✓		
Spain			✓	
Sweden			✓	
UK			✓	

No country has guidelines with regard to best practice. In Finland and Denmark, the doctor is legally required to inform the patient of the diagnosis, and does so. Although this is a legal requirement in Germany, it does not always occur in practice. In most countries, the doctor usually informs the family, and sometimes the patient, depending on the stage of illness and the doctor's judgement with regard to the patient's capacity to understand the information.

There appears to be some association between the stage of development of dementia care and the doctor's willingness to disclose the diagnosis to the patient, suggesting that as practice improves and the diagnosis is made earlier, patients are more likely to be informed. With the availability of new treatments, early diagnosis will become more important and be demanded by the patient and family, and this may accelerate changes in disclosure practice.

Adoption of new treatments for AD

Within the past three years, cholinesterase inhibitors (CIs) have become widely available for the symptomatic treatment of mild AD. The evidence for their use in treatment is that approximately 30% of patients may show a symptomatic improvement in terms of cognition and function in clinical trials. The real-life effect of such treatment is still emerging. Supporters of CIs argue that these treatments are worthwhile because they may delay institutionalisation, thereby saving costs. However, prolonging illness duration with increased indirect and direct costs for patient maintenance in a community setting may not translate into real financial savings and may only transfer costs back to families. Although only recently approved and available in Europe, a review of CI availability, and the pattern of their prescription, sheds some light on the challenges faced when research developments are transmitted into clinical practice in the dementia care arena.

The ETAS study ascertained that CIs are now approved in all European countries. However, even in countries where they are approved for use, their availability can be restricted by budgetary constraints and fewer patients than expected are actually prescribed these agents. Their availability for prescription by specialist or GP is not consistent throughout Europe. In some countries it is specialists only who can prescribe (Austria). In others, only the first prescription must be by a specialist (Italy, France) and in others (Ireland, Sweden), any doctor can prescribe. Given the current state of expertise regarding detection and diagnosis, the decision to allow GPs unrestricted prescribing would appear premature. However, issues of drug costs and budgets, rather than the level of clinical expertise and acumen may have more to do with this issue.

Conclusions: where are the gaps and how to fill them?

The ETAS study has provided useful qualitative comparative information regarding clinical practice with respect to dementia care across

Europe. A number of common issues emerge which point to gaps in the system that must be addressed in policy initiatives within each country and across the EU.

Poor assessment procedures in primary care

Improving the assessment and diagnosis of dementia is a challenge that is common to all countries. Access to any care system should begin with appropriate detection and diagnosis. Patients, and their care-givers, need access to appropriate assessment in order to receive care. But by the same token, patients should not access care without appropriate assessment and diagnosis. At present, many sufferers, particularly at an early stage, are not detected, or are detected too late to be able to receive a meaningful intervention. A major challenge for primary care across Europe is to increase awareness regarding detection and diagnosis and to bring about the routine use of cognitive screening tools and assessments that accurately detect and reflect dementia patients' *silent disability*. Public education regarding the early symptoms of dementia will also be important to improve detection, by encouraging individuals and their carers to present to general practitioners at an earlier stage of the disease process. However, as suggested in Chapter 4, there are some legal disincentives to doing this.

Specialists in practice: getting them and getting the right balance

Specialists can play a crucial role in the development of practice in a particular country. Where dementia care is at an early stage of development there is invariably little specialisation. A response to this situation would be to support and foster specialists' development, so that they can act as advocates of good clinical practice. Almost two-thirds of countries examined had no accreditation for geriatric psychiatry. This specialty traditionally deals with behavioural disturbances in dementia and this aspect of care and practice can potentially suffer or remain under-developed without it. While specialists' leadership is clearly important in its own right, collaboration and co-operation between and across specialties is also vital if a seamless and patient-centred dementia practice is to be developed.

Improving the image of dementia in practice

Dementia generally has a negative image. Professionals take a nihilistic view, and there is a sense that identifying the disease does not help the problem. This may be exacerbated by the fact that there is often a dearth of services available for the patient and carer, and this acts as a brake on earlier diagnosis and possible intervention. A challenge to educators and trainers is to reverse this image problem. Education must begin early in training.

Perhaps the most sobering finding from the ETAS review is the dearth of empirical data regarding clinical practice throughout Europe. What evidence is available indicates that assessment techniques are poor in primary care and that few patients have a dementia work-up. To address clinical practice issues across Europe it would be helpful to derive empirical evidence of the current practice in each country. This would further highlight the gaps and encourage development.

References

1 Bayer AJ, Pathy MSJ and Twining C (1987) The memory clinic: a new approach to the detection of early dementia. *Drugs.* **33**(2): 84–9.

2 Larson EB (1998) Recognition of dementia: discovering the silent epidemic. *J Am Geriatr Soc.* **46**(12): 1576–7.

3 Fraser RM and Healy R (1986) Psychogeriatric liaison: a service to a district general hospital. *Bull R Coll Psychiatrists.* **10**: 312–14.

4 Stoppe G, Sandholzer H and Staedt J (1996) Cerebral cognitive deficits in the aged. Diagnostic and therapeutic standards: organisation of strategies for problem detection and solution. *Z Arztl Fortbild (Jena).* **90**.

5 Stoppe G, Sandholzer H, Staedt J *et al.* (1995) Reasons for prescribing cognition enhancers in primary care: results of a representative survey in Lower Saxony, Germany. *Int J Clin Pharmacol Ther.* **33**: 486–90.

6 Valenciano R, Morera A, Rodriguez-Perera F *et al.* (1989) Diagnosis of dementia in primary care. *Arch Neurobiol (Madr).* **52**: 174–7.

7 Alzheimer's Disease Society (1995) *Right From the Start: primary healthcare and dementia.* Alzheimer's Disease Society, London.

8   Wolf, LE, Woods JP and Reid J (1995) Do general practitioners and old age psychiatrists differ in their attitude to dementia. *Int J Ger Psych.* **10**: 66–9.

9   Warner M, Furnish S, Lawlor B *et al.* (1998) *European Transnational Alzheimer Study (ETAS).* Welsh Institute for Health and Social Care, Pontypridd.

10 Drickamer MA and Lachs MS (1992) Should patients with Alzheimer's disease be told their diagnosis? *NEJM.* **326**: 947–54.

11 Rice K and Warner N (1994) Breaking the bad news: what do psychiatrists tell patients with dementia about their illness? *Int J Ger Psych.* **9**: 467–71.

12 Maguire JP, Kirby M, Coen R *et al.* (1996) Family member's attitudes toward telling the patient with Alzheimer's Disease their diagnosis. *BMJ.* **313**: 529–30.

13 Vassilas CA and Donaldson J (1998) Telling the truth – what do general practitioners say to patients with dementia? *Br J Gen Pract.* **48**: 1081–2.

7

Developing support worker training programmes for Alzheimer's care provided at home

Christine Flori and Michel Aberlen

Introduction

Provision of home care has not yet succeeded in becoming a general reality, either in terms of support worker training or for elderly neuro-degenerative patients. The family remains the largest provider of *care*, followed by neighbours and organised voluntary groups – for instance pensioner associations. The input of support workers is therefore needed when the more professional resources already in place appear limited or insufficient.

It should be remembered that people suffering from these disorders need assistance not because they are socially maladjusted but because they are ill. Training should aim to address the specific needs of the illnesses, in order to help families feel confident in reclaiming some social and psychological space for themselves. This also requires suitable accommodation and services to be available for the sufferer when the family can no longer cope, and a deliberate policy to help the family feel less guilty and enable them to step back for a while if necessary. It is essential, therefore, to introduce support workers who have been trained to meet the needs of families as well as the needs of patients. Both require an awareness of the need for dignity, citizenship and a humane existence.

A study of a number of European countries shows that the 'social' professions find themselves responsible for caring.[1] However, the person with dementia also has a set of 'medical' needs stemming from their illness, and it is important that generic support staff are aware of these and have support from professionals to identify them. Moreover, helpers often have to cope with the bad temper, depression, loss of will and dementia of someone who cannot take (or express) decisions any more, even though they fully remain a *person* with their own past history and life history. Again, *professional* back-up is crucial.

Support worker skills required

These are wide-ranging. The helper needs to know not only *what* to do, but also *how* to do it. The need frequently encountered in general geriatric care – not only with Alzheimer's patients but also with other senile elderly patients – is for communication training.

In order for carers to be able to adequately support someone with memory loss, speech disorder and behaviour disorder (aggression, apathy or mood disorder), they should be trained to interpret the disorder as it occurs, especially where the appropriate response is not of a medical nature. This can be a major challenge for support workers who are usually, up to this time, only asked to do more mundane tasks such as shopping, housework or washing.

The worker's role will be to enhance the patient's abilities, taking care of the sufferer, but through engagement. It is important that the sufferer should be clean, well-dressed and mobile, but helpers should be able to go further. An Alzheimer's patient taken back into a normal home situation is often able to regain significant abilities well beyond the expectations of many professional carers. In addition, sufferers still feel emotion – affection, happiness, sorrow and creativity – and can become bored. The helper, together with the family when there is one, should be trained to counteract the more negative tendencies.

The skills required cross the boundaries of several disciplines and must be focused on an individual who often has disabilities of comprehension. The support worker must know how to achieve the respect of sufferer and family, at the same time as providing care. Home-based care-givers also work in very different conditions from those encountered by the health and social care teams in hospitals or in a medical environment. They cannot avoid facing the family on their own territory, making the context in which they work sometimes quite difficult. In this environment it is essential that the helper's role is defined in agreement with the family, immediately after diagnosis but before attendance at the patient's home.

Training dimensions

The help to be provided to sufferers and their families starts very early. First, the person with Alzheimer's disease (AD) can be helped by an early diagnosis, and thus support workers must take note of any information from the family that can be collected and passed on to social and medical workers. Consequently, it is vital to think about the necessity of training in the area of observation. Following this, support offered to the AD sufferer remains essential. Indeed, during the time when the patient still has a certain degree of autonomy, support adapted to their individual needs can be provided in order to prevent rapid degeneration.

Developed countries suffer from a great tendency towards service compartmentalisation, and healthcare staff rarely interact effectively with those from social care. Thus the work of support workers must be supplemented with nurses and nursing auxiliaries who can undertake domiciliary treatments. Throughout, the support workers will:

- be aware of the totality and complexity of the issues
- consider the ways they will work within the family environment and
- develop their own approach, since every sufferer is different.

In general terms, support workers must have a strong sense of identity in order to be able to work alongside the other professional carers in a real partnership. They should work in a way that encourages appropriate autonomy and responsibility.

The main skills offered within current training courses

These are summarised in Table 7.1(a)–(c) and should be mastered by the support worker by the end of training. The main thrust is that the support worker should be able:

- to take appropriate actions within a legal, institutional and ethical context as regards the patient, the family and themselves

Table 7.1: Training requirements for support workers – a general European picture

(a) Across all areas

1 Ageing process	2 Observing	3 Caring/ maintaining	4 Participation	5 Helping/ answering	6 Encouraging	7 Communicating
In relation to the patient, the family; according to ethics legal and institutional problems – his/her level of self-support – his/her feelings His/her responsibilities To create a relationship based on confidence – to respect privacy – to respect the culture of the patient To be able to adapt to different situations	Sleep rhythm and factors influencing sleep – problems of mobility and balance – listening to wishes, needs, complaints – relations to treatments, disability – resources Changes in health – in behaviour Loss of appetite, thirst	Respecting individuality – pressure sores – diet – prescription – incontinence – body temperature – immobility – behaviour – delirium, depression, hallucination Atmosphere, morale	Organising meals – preventing incontinence – adaptation of timetable and environment to needs for rest and peace – team working	Aggression – negative reactions – feelings of fear – wandering Buying – managing, preparing meals Acting in case of emergency	Facilitation of adapted activities – social relations – communication – stimulating remaining capacities	Pressure sores – noting temperature – mobility problems, balance – communicating with patient, relations and family, social services, other services Relations with the elderly person at the end of his life – in case of death or bereavement

(b) In relation to the patient

1 Ageing process	2 Observing	3 Caring/maintaining	4 Participation	5 Helping/answering	6 Encouraging	7 Communicating
Rights – respect for privacy	Temperature	Care comfort – hazardous situations – risks of pressure sores – body temperature – lack of mobility Good morale	Overcoming difficult situations	Treatment – comfort Aggression – negative reactions – feeling of fear Wandering	Communication – participation in daily life and leisure activities – facilitation of adapted activities	

(c) In relation to the family/environment

1 Ageing process	2 Observing	3 Caring/maintaining	4 Participation	5 Helping/answering	6 Encouraging	7 Communicating
Daily needs Organisation Legislation	Resources	Relations within the family	Ergonomic improvements – organisation – diet – adaptation of timetable and environment to needs of rest and peace		Communication – visits – adapted activities	Hygiene – aesthetics – clothing – risk of pressure sores – problems of mobility – of balance In case of death – bereavement

- to notice the patterns underlying the daily life of the patient and his family
- to anticipate/maintain the health, the activity and the harmony of both the family and the patient
- to participate with the family, the relatives or a team in an overall strategy, organising and adapting to fit in with daily life
- to look for/provide appropriate responses to specific situations
- to stimulate/undertake psychosocial activity and
- to communicate within a multi-relational framework.

A general observation is that the training programmes lead towards being able to provide generic assistance, responding to the needs of older people across the board; specialist attention to neuro-degenerative disease problems is lacking. To correct this, many training organisations now train support workers, volunteers and families, not through open meetings, but on an individual basis for particular carers and their families. In other instances, they gather together the experience of the various carers, particularly those of families and professionals, thus helping to define the limits and the complementary nature of the support workers' own specialised activities. Such approaches to training are obviously a useful development.

Guidelines for the training of support workers across Europe

It is important to develop a coherent and cohesive approach across Europe which takes into account the requirements identified above. Many thousands of people require training!

The task will not be easy. In May 1995, at the 6th Conference of Ministers in charge of Social Security in Lisbon, the member states had some problems finding a common definition for *dependence*. Some countries included the notion of *handicap* within that of *dependence*. At the end of that meeting, the 34 member states of the European Council delivered a common definition and agreed to give special attention to the training of those in charge of the care of dependent people. In February 1996, a report on AD and the prevention of cognitive function disorders for elderly people was presented to the European Parliament.[2] This was followed by a resolution, unanimously adopted, which asked the Commission to present a programme of action to fight against AD and connected syndromes, while the member states should:

- define an appropriate strategy and take measures accordingly, particularly with regard to co-operation between social services and health services
- promote the organisation of training courses specifically aimed at paramedical personnel.

Many carers have attended some training courses, mainly thanks to voluntary associations which are often more accessible than the official system. For the last ten years, the increased need for home care provision to elderly people, representing an average of 60–70% of people using services, has led to a modification of the nature of home care. It has lost its aim of being temporary care and has become seen as long-term. It is now more technical, and consequently requires personnel to be increasingly qualified. As a result, the status of home care personnel has been redefined and the question of their training has been specifically addressed for the first time.

Initial training is a prerequisite. This does not exist in all countries, and where it does, it is rarely sufficient to meet demand because of cost constraints. The variation between countries stems in large part from the absence of consensus among personnel doing the same work. Moreover, there are few formal linkages between the different categories of home care personnel. The training offered allows the carer's daily work to act as the focus for their development, but it appears that the content of training varies, as everyone has different experiences, habits and preferences. Thus different observers across the EU have reported on general medical practitioners' ignorance about the treatment of older people generally, and particularly those suffering from dementia. This also regularly applies to social workers (employed by councils or hospitals) working in people's homes and support workers.

From the beginning, the European Community set up systems to compare and recognise qualifications between the different countries. These caused many technical problems and difficulties were faced in finding common definitions for countries which have neither the same economic structures, nor the same systems for employment training and classification. The very notion of qualification does not have the same meaning in each country. The support of the European authorities for improving equivalence between qualifications was motivated by the desire to increase workforce mobility (which, however, remains limited).

Various studies show that a consensus on codification and validation of qualifications is more likely to succeed when people from a work sector discuss the conditions within each country and address each specific context. The issues concerning the consequences of change are taken into account in the training and qualification systems. Another approach consists of defining professional profiles – this aims to make it easier to assess qualifications by creating a common description of work activities and professional skills that corresponds to a particular function, rather than to a profession or an occupation.

These various pressures indicate a continuing need to carry on thinking about common concepts of skills development and the construction of qualification systems. As far as elderly people suffering from neuro-degenerative disease are concerned, the function of the carer must be definitely recognised. Indeed, it might be desirable to reach a common concept of the very notion of qualification. It should:

- be composed of all skills gathered by an individual, not only through training, but also through personal and professional experience
- not only be the result of educational learning leading to a diploma, but also be subject to continuous development throughout life
- recognise that knowledge and know-how can also be developed in the working situation
- involve governments and the work sector in its construction.

In areas involving carers of people suffering from neuro-degenerative disease, whose working conditions are far from stabilised, a European debate will build an important reference point for structuring within each country. Furthermore, considering the increasing importance of the debates all around Europe on the training curriculum and the conditions in which the diplomas should be awarded, European co-operation in this area will influence the long-term evolution of training systems.

Creating common references for health support workers raises many issues beyond those relating to the inventory of skills to be set up in each country. The debates between countries should deal with the conditions in which skills are acquired and knowledge in this area is recognised. It is not certain that even the countries in the SEDI partnership will find common answers to all these issues.[1] The quality of information exchange within Europe on this topic depends above all on the capacity to create the conditions necessary for co-operation between governments, and on the ability to make progress, in a methodical way, on the specific concerns identified.

Beyond this, it is important at the micro-level to create the prospect of a professional career for carers, with specialisation remaining possible to encourage further career progression. On a macro-economic level, to have a comprehensive system of well-trained home carers would cost less than caring for an increasing number of patients in institutions, where they would have to be placed if they could not stay at home.

Conclusions

It is now a matter of urgency to start building a network of skills and find common qualification guidelines within Europe, which look beyond national interests and the carers' status within each member state.

One way forward could be to insist on families explaining their requirements. Another way would be to recognise the skills of home support workers in the short term, and in the medium term, to give them career prospects.

Developing training in home support care for patients suffering from neuro-degenerative disorders represents a social challenge, a human necessity, an ethical priority and a potential opening up of new practices and new jobs at the European level. This makes it necessary to gather and exchange ideas in order to help build a European vision which will take into account the economic, social, cultural and psychological aspects specific to each country.

The setting up of training adapted to the specific needs of each country, but relying on a plurality of methods, can only contribute to the reinforcement of social, cultural and ethical links within the European Union. The quality of life and medical, social and psychological care of patients with neuro-degenerative diseases will also be improved.

References

1   Moulias G (1997) *Study of Alzheimer's Disease Support in Germany, France, Italy, Great Britain, Portugal and Sweden*. SEDI, Paris.

2   Presented by M Danilo Poggiolini, February 1996.

8

Disseminating information on Alzheimer's disease to European stakeholders

David McDaid, Jean Georges and
Leen Meulenberg

Introduction

While much research effort is concentrated on understanding the different aspects of Alzheimer's disease (AD) – physiological, psychological and social – the impact and adoption of new therapies will be dependent, to a considerable degree, upon dissemination of information to healthcare professionals and other formal care-givers. More and more, the emphasis is on evidence-based care. Family care-givers, as a particularly vulnerable group, also require information about the disease itself and about services which they can access, in order to be able to respond to problems they may face from time to time.

This chapter sets out to address information issues, examining the importance of dissemination strategies and identifying the knowledge requirements of different target audiences. It provides some examples of how information on AD is moved across the European Union and elsewhere, identifying shortcomings in this process. Finally, it considers the long-term implications of improved access to information, particularly in view of new technological developments.

Gaps in knowledge

Medical personnel and social care workers should have most information on the clinical effects and consequences for carers and patients, but many have insufficient training given that psycho-geriatrics is a relatively new specialty and AD a new specialist area. General practitioners, for instance, may have limited exposure to AD: in Denmark, for example, less than 10% of those with dementia have a medical examination, and this has been attributed, in part, to a lack of knowledge amongst both primary healthcare practitioners and the general public.[1]

There is considerable responsibility, therefore, to help empower caregivers and patients to make informed choices about appropriate care and assistance. But despite the reported importance of information for caregivers, studies have repeatedly reported that a structured, personalised and systematised approach to the provision of information is the exception rather than the rule.[2,3]

Much of the reported work thus far comes from the UK. In rural England, 70% of carers felt they required additional information and advice, and subsequently an information booklet was reported to be helpful to 87% of them.[4] In another survey, commissioned by the UK Carers' National Association, of carers coming into contact with the NHS, respondents were asked about their experiences in receiving both general information on caring and medical information about the person they were caring for. Only 40% were informed about respite services, 20% about legal rights and entitlements and 11% about any training that might be available.[5] This study also found that 64% did not know of any information that would be helpful that could be obtained from general practitioners' surgeries. This suggested that their GPs either did not have access to information on local services, or were unaware of the benefits of providing it. Similarly, in a survey from the Spanish Ministry of Social Work, regions in the south of the country were found to be much less well informed about domiciliary care services than those elsewhere. 84% of GPs in Andalucia and 67% in the regions of Castilla – La Mancha, Murcia and Extramedura – did not know anything at all about such services.[6]

The impact of dissemination (or lack of it) can also be illustrated by considering the use of day care centres in Catalonia and the Basque country. These regions of Spain have the highest number of available places per head of population. In Catalonia, where the centres have been well publicised, demand has outstripped supply. By contrast, in the Basque country, a lack of publicity can be associated with low demand for places, with a recent survey finding that over 70% of people receiving domiciliary assistance were unaware of the existence of day care centres.[6]

The ethical implications of increasing access to information cannot be ignored. Care-givers may not want the opportunity to make choices, preferring instead to leave all decision making in the hands of health and social care professionals. They may find decision making stressful, feeling they do not have enough time to make informed decisions or not wishing to be responsible for the consequences. Beyond this, raising the profile of treatments for AD, which have been shown thus far to have only minimal success, can take resources away from proven interventions for care-givers and patients.

Information requirements

Having identified some of the gaps in knowledge and the need for information, the specific requirements of different groups are now outlined.

Policy-makers

A prime requirement for this group is the collation of information on the incidence and prevalence of AD. This can be difficult to do. One survey of GPs in Scotland found, for example, that only 31% of respondents kept identifiable records of people with dementia.[7] Another requirement is to have information on the current provision of health and social care resources and their utilisation, to help in determining the future supply of services that will be required.

In Catalonia, for example, the National Health Plan recognised AD as a special health problem and began to collect information as a priority from 1996. This was seen as the first step in creating a database for both professionals and care-givers. Greater co-ordination of communication between medical and social care professionals has also been emphasised as a policy objective in Catalonia.[6]

In Lombardy, in northern Italy, the Plan Alzheimer Lombardia was commissioned to develop an integrated approach, and nine regional Alzheimer centres were established. The prime purpose of these centres is to provide information and training to families and the public in order to increase awareness and minimise risks.[8] Another initiative is the telephone helpline for care-givers in Denmark, supported by the Danish Ministry of Social Affairs.[9] At the European level, a number of research projects on ADRD have been funded by the European Commission.

The provision of high quality accessible information, coupled with other community-based services, may be cost-effective for health and social care funders in delaying institutionalisation of patients. Support from formal services may also allow care-givers to maintain employment and social networks.

The public also requires data on the relative merits of different treatment and management options. In the UK and the Netherlands, for example, specific funding has been made available through national health technology assessment bodies to determine the clinical efficacy and cost-effectiveness of dementia-related drugs and cognitive therapies. The National Institute for Clinical Excellence (NICE) in England and Wales is currently appraising pharmaceutical therapies for dementia. Conferences sponsored by national governments and local/regional policy-makers, such as in Ireland, France and Sweden, have exchanged information and stimulated many debates.

Health and social care professionals

Primary care practitioners have to deal with a broad range of ailments and cannot easily be as well informed in specialist areas such as AD. Education, training and basic information on the diagnosis and management of dementia are required. In a survey of GPs in the UK, 71% of 691 responding felt inadequately prepared on AD, despite the fact that two-thirds had undergone some training in psycho-geriatrics.[10] This survey also reported that only 14% of GPs referred care-givers to their local Alzheimer's disease society group, believing that to do so was not their responsibility.

Education and training can help break down unfavourable attitudes within the medical profession. Practitioners need to be aware that early diagnosis and referral may not only provide care-givers and patients with more time to prepare for the future, as well as slowing the onset of the illness, but may also help to identify those carers and patients who would benefit from support. Measures such as the introduction in the UK of mandatory annual health checks for the over-75s may increase the likelihood that practitioners come into contact and recognise people with probable AD. However, one Scottish study reported that general practitioners found little value in the early disclosure of a diagnosis of dementia, believing the problem to be largely social. Specialists, by contrast, were more likely to provide information to patients and care-givers, and believed the issues arising to be both medical and social.[11]

Professional guidelines can be used to disseminate best practice and influence attitudes; but they are more likely to have an impact if formulated through expert consensus by peer groups, alongside consultation with local practitioners and care-giver associations.[12] In Sweden, for example, national guidelines on diagnostic criteria have been published by a consensus group in the official journal of the Swedish Medical Association, although it is reported that they are rarely used outside dementia research clinics.[13] The German Association of General Practitioners has produced a 'Dementia Manual' containing guidelines on therapy for patients with AD, which includes pharmaceutical, cognitive and social issues.[14] In the Netherlands, the Dutch General Practitioners' Society has published guidelines in co-operation with care-givers, which provide background information on AD and advice on care, treatments and problems that care-givers will encounter.[15]

Wimo has suggested that social care authorities require further action to develop their own education plans to educate staff.[16] These professionals must be especially aware of the difficulties carers may have in expressing need for help, particularly as the disease progresses and social isolation increases. They should be sensitive to the emotional state of care-givers when disclosing information, as they may be in denial about AD in a loved one, or hide difficulties that they have in coping.[17] Greater awareness of the broad needs of people with AD and their care-givers will focus the co-ordinated efforts of medical and social care support services

Care-givers and people with AD

Care-givers will require access to information on many issues – particularly about understanding the clinical prognosis, symptoms and the limitations of treatments. This may help care-givers and people with possible AD to recognise when to consult with physicians. As AD is a distressing subject, information must be conveyed in a tactful and supportive manner. If an early diagnosis of dementia is made, then they also require counselling and support to help them accept their situation and plan for the future.

Many care-givers do not come to the attention of formal agencies until their inability to cope becomes obvious. This may be due to a lack of information about services, and can also be exacerbated through geographical inaccessibility and the various other factors which prevent the equitable provision of health and other services. Those who live in such areas as northern Sweden and the Scottish Highlands may well not come to the attention of formal or voluntary agencies until in a very advanced stage of the condition. Additionally, they are also likely to have reduced general access to all services, including information, due to the increased costs of provision in rural communities.[18]

There are a number of areas where information is vital.

- Advice on legal affairs and entitlements to financial benefits – extra stress and expense may be encountered by care-givers and sufferers if the necessary legal arrangements are not put in place in a timely fashion.
- Unnecessary hardship may be endured if financial benefits go unclaimed, particularly where care-givers have had to give up or reduce their employment assistance and advice may be required with complex forms.
- Education and training can help care-givers to cope with everyday living, for example providing advice on how to lift, dress and stimulate people with AD.

Ready access to information from voluntary groups and trained counsellors, providing both advice and emotional support, provides reassurance for care-givers, and can significantly reduce the stress levels associated with caring.[2] Innovative mechanisms for communication, such as telephone helplines and Internet chat forums, may in themselves provide some form of respite, helping to create virtual social networks to complement support from family and friends. The CANDID dementia chat forum, maintained by the Dementia Research Group at the Institute of Neurology in London, provides one example of the opportunity for care-givers to talk with professionals, in strict confidence, whilst maintaining their anonymity if they wish.[20]

The public

It is important to overcome the public reticence to discuss AD if ageism, fear and common misconceptions are to be tackled. The value of *care-giving* to society should also be promoted. An increase in general awareness and understanding of AD may encourage care-givers – and individuals who suspect that they might have dementia – to approach formal agencies at an earlier stage. This may increase the workload faced by already stretched formal services: for example, the use of a dementia telephone helpline in Scotland peaked following a voluntary organisation's annual dementia awareness week; and a conference in Belgium was oversubscribed following a poster campaign in prominent public locations. But from the voluntary agency's perspective, generating awareness is also a vital means of raising revenue.

Existing and emerging media for the dissemination of information on AD

Technology has increased the range of media that are available to disseminate information on AD to particular audiences. Alongside traditional approaches such as books, training courses, journal articles, leaflets and fundraising events, innovations such as telephone helplines, specialist expert centres, intranets and web pages are now increasingly used to raise awareness. This section provides examples of their use in Europe and their potential to impact on target audiences.

The Internet

The Internet potentially offers a highly effective mechanism for information distribution. It can be used for direct communication through email and 'virtual chatting' as well as for access to documentation and audio-visual materials. At present, most documents are accessed via the World Wide Web using software which can be cheaply installed on personal computers. This presents several advantages over traditional paper documents. First, they can be updated easily at short notice to incorporate the latest information; second, they can present vast quantities of information which otherwise would be bulky and expensive to print; and third, their format allows users to search and access information on topics of interest.

The Internet can also help to reach carers who are geographically and socially isolated, or feel that meetings and brochures are not adequate for their individual needs.[19] It can also potentially help minority groups. For example, Alzheimer Europe provides information in all major languages spoken in the European Union, and some web pages in the UK provide information in languages such as Bengali and Urdu. A number of well-developed sites in Europe are listed in Box 8.1.

Box 8.1: Examples of websites

Alzheimer Europe: http://www.alzheimer-europe.org/
Alzheimer Scotland: http://www.alzscot.org/
Dementia Association of Sweden: http://www.demensforbundet.se/
European Alzheimer Clearing House: http://www.each.be
University of Stirling Dementia Services Development Centre:
   http://www.stir.ac.uk/Departments/HumanSciences/dsdc/
Italian Alzheimer Web: http://www.italz.it/

These provide a wealth of information on publications, forthcoming conferences, seminars, ongoing research projects and how to access specialist services. Websites are also extremely useful for handling enquiries from non-care-givers, particularly in the voluntary sector, where staff may be restricted, allowing organisations at local level to spend more time assisting those who require the most help. The medium is well adapted to answering general enquiries for information in a rapid and low cost way.

The ITALZ web page in Italy, for example, aims to collect all information resources available in Italian, to help sufferers and care-givers, as well as researchers, students and medical staff. It also has an electronic mailing list to inform subscribers of the latest developments, conference announcements and to act as a forum for queries and the exchange of information. A number of documents can be downloaded on a wide range of topics to assist care-givers and people with AD. Users can click on a detailed map to obtain information on services available throughout the country. Regional maps are then displayed, as in the example in Figure 8.1, which shows Bergamo in Lombardia, and data is displayed about the local Alzheimer association and the activities of a specialist medical centre.

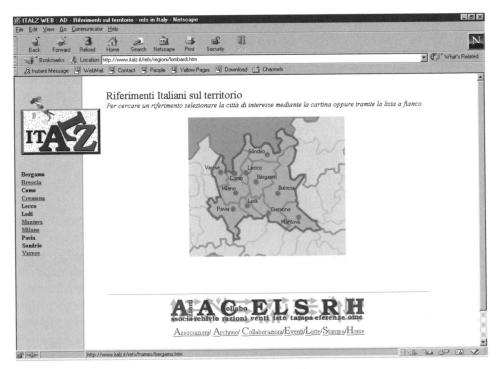

Figure 8.1:   Accessing information from the ITALZ website.

In addition, the medium is increasingly used by other formal bodies. In the UK, many hospitals and local authorities publicise their services on the World Wide Web. One example is the Norfolk County Council web page in England (http://www.norfolk.gov.uk/), which includes detailed information on help available from social services, as well as links to support from voluntary agencies such as Crossroads.

A wide range of other groups also use the Web. Academic institutions use the medium to publicise ongoing research and conferences with which they are involved, and as a means of disseminating discussion papers. The pharmaceutical industry has invested in professionally-designed websites which contain not only information about products but also other general information as well. National governments publish policy papers, reports and other information. For example, in the UK, the Department of Social Security's site has information on benefits which are available to people with AD and care-givers; and in Ireland, the Department of Health provides information on entitlements to healthcare services in general for the elderly.

One innovation now becoming more common is the 'chat forum', which allows individuals to communicate in real time via the Internet. Care-givers' forums have been set up to seek financial and other support, and the net also provides access to expert assistance, as with the CANDID dementia care-givers' forum based in the UK, where a specialist in dementia participates in discussions at specified times.[20] Group email is also used by care-givers, academics and professionals to ask questions, publicise events and activities and discuss aspects of dementia case management. Responses are posted to the entire group or just to the individual who sent the original message.

Intranets

Although using the same technology as the Internet, intranets are *closed* systems, with access limited to those with an appropriate registration and password. Users are assigned different levels of access to information and a high degree of confidentiality is maintained.

One such system is being developed by Alzheimer Europe to exchange information, initially between members of Alzheimer associations and professionals. This is to be collected nationally and then made available from the centre. By making the system available to both professionals and associations, it is hoped the database will be used to advise patients and care-givers of help that is available from local Alzheimer's disease associations. The system will also provide access to information from pharmaceutical companies on the use of medication. This would not be limited to specific AD drugs, but would also contain information on other relevant therapies such as antidepressants.

Specifically, Alzheimer Europe arrangements will contain the following:

- Alzheimer Europe documentation
- schedule of forthcoming meetings, conferences and symposia
- publications and other information published by associations
- addresses and contacts for national/regional associations
- day care centres, sitting services, domiciliary and respite care services, etc.
- pharmaceutical information on existing and new drugs and drug trials
- chat forum.

A well-structured system such as this can be an invaluable database to aid telephone helpline operators when on 'live' calls, although this would depend on the speed of the Internet. The ability to restrict access to certain information may help to answer some of the ethical problems caused by disseminating information among a wide audience. Conversely, however, the need for a password may actually reduce the use by the target audience unless mechanisms are in place to assist people who forget their passwords.

Telephone helplines

Telephone helplines – like the Internet – are a useful way of providing information and advice to care-givers, who, in particular, are unable to attend support group meetings due to geographical or social isolation. They are run by a number of Alzheimer associations and other voluntary groups in Europe.

One such is from Alzheimer Scotland – Action on Dementia which provides free access to information and emotional support, 24 hours a day, all year for people with dementia, their care-givers, relatives, friends and professionals. Their aim is to empower callers by providing them with appropriate contacts and information to help them make their own choices.

In 1996/1997, 2605 calls were received by the helpline, peaking at the time of Dementia Awareness Week. Two-thirds were from care-givers, with a further 19% from professionals or students; but 4% of calls were from people who had a diagnosis of, or suspected they had, dementia. More than 50% of calls were specifically on caring issues, and 35%

wanted emotional support. Other issues included long-term care, community care services, legal advice and financial help. A survey of callers to the helpline found that 96% felt the information they received was very useful and 90% stated that they would contact the helpline again. When asked what they had expected, 85% said information, 58% advice, 27% emotional support and 24% to be put in contact with practical help. Training of those manning the systems is critical in the light of this.[21]

Whilst the helpline is clearly useful to callers, Alzheimer Scotland estimates that it currently reaches only 8% of all care-givers, and other contact strategies are required: this is particularly relevant when it is necessary to disseminate up-to-date information on drug therapies.

Specialist dementia centres

Specialist multidisciplinary centres also provide opportunities to disseminate information and increase awareness among professional groups. One such, the Dementia Services Development Centre (DSDC) at the University of Stirling, in Scotland, has a dedicated information service, including a specialist library where both bibliographic and service databases are compiled. Extensive information is also available through the centre's website.

The DSDC also organises regular workshops and seminars aimed at 'extending and improving services to people with dementia and their carers'.[22] These events cover many different topics. For example, the 1999 programme included workshops on art therapy, complementary medicine, housing and support for people with dementia, non-verbal communication and new methods for conveying messages to people with dementia. A training service is available, geared towards providing learning opportunities for staff who are working in the formal and charitable sectors. In addition, the centre has also produced a number of training publications and developed specialised training projects.

A variation of the specialist centre is a clearing house identifying high quality and appropriate information relevant to a range of different groups. The principal example of this is the Belgian-based European Alzheimer Clearing House (EACH) which aims to collect, analyse, compile, disseminate and promote the application of:

* knowledge of AD and related disorders
* successful management approaches for patients, families, care-givers, administrators, decision makers and the general public and
* evidence-based care to achieve the highest possible quality of life for patients and their families.

The goals of EACH are to contribute to:

- developing a more integrated, non-fragmented approach
- increasing public awareness in order to improve services
- a higher quality of life for patients and their families
- providing empowerment of self-help and policy development
- making available a better alignment between EU member states' activities and some form of European norms.

In order to do this, a consortium was organised which included a network of formal and informal care-giver organisations, policy-makers, professional bodies and research centres. Information on priority projects across EU countries is objectively analysed with the assistance of recognised national experts and international networks. Priority topics include:

- training for professionals and non-professionals
- good care practice
- information exchange for Alzheimer associations
- socio-economic impact of AD
- ethical issues
- support programmes for sufferers and carers
- nursing qualifications
- substance counselling
- clinical activities.

A dissemination strategy has been developed by EACH with the help of experts, including the media. Audiences for specific information are identified, and then information is published, using one or more approaches to maximise impact. Methods include producing workbooks, training manuals and brochures for professionals and carers, as well as providing access to online databases and other information on the Internet.

Three specific databases are under development by EACH. The first listing, of European services, aims to provide information on the addresses and contacts for good practice in different types of AD care within specific regions of a country. For example, selecting Scotland gives access to material on best practice in nursing home care, weekend day care, day care and specialist care for those with early onset dementia. A second database provides information on the different Alzheimer associations in Europe, their publications, and other services they might provide, such as day care, web pages and telephone helplines. The third database will provide information on different substances that may be associated with AD, such as new pharmaceutical products, nutritional substances and toxic substances.

Conclusions

This chapter has illustrated ways in which improved access to, and use of, information should be considered an essential component both for improving the management of AD by professionals, and for policy-makers as they consider resource allocation. Access to a wide range of appropriate information also helps empower both care-givers and patients in making informed choices. Access to information in Europe is at present haphazard, and in particular, many care-givers may not be aware of entitlements to basic services and financial assistance. How-ever, getting information to care-givers and patients already known to the formal services is only one part of the equation; reaching uniden-tified care-givers can only be done through measures that target the general public.

Primary care practitioners have a pivotal role to play where they are the first point of contact. Physicians and nurses need to be aware of the needs of both care-givers and patients and this will only happen through increasing the amount of formal training in medical and nursing education and through provision of incentives to attend high quality continuing education courses. Even where GPs have had some training in psycho-geriatrics, this may have included little on the needs of care-givers. Importantly, if new anti-dementia drugs are to be used effectively, medical professionals need information on how to recognise early signs of dementia in their patients. One way to achieve this could be the creation of regional centres of excellence specialising in AD, pro-viding continuing training for health and social care workers. This would also increase the number of specialists available to whom referrals could be made.

New technology will increasingly have an important role to play, but should be complementary to, rather than a replacement for, traditional ways of passing information. Effective use of the existing approaches to informing care-givers is essential. Ideally, this should occur in a number of ways: either face to face or by telephone and through access to leaflets. Written materials should be jargon-free, available in large print and in minority languages. No assumptions should be made about knowledge that users have of support services.

The Internet is now widely used across Europe for providing infor-mation on AD. Increasingly, journals are producing electronic versions, and medical databases and guidelines can be accessed online. Health and social care services can co-ordinate their activities through electronic communication and care-givers may obtain access to information confi-dentially and at a time of their own choosing.

Some caution, however, must be exercised about over-estimating the impact and use of the Internet. A major difficulty will be defining what is meant by quality. Websites from specialist centres, organisations such as EACH and patient/care-giver associations like Alzheimer Europe, will need a high profile, being designed carefully to ensure that they are easily found, contain accurate information and can retain credibility.

Furthermore, as care-givers become more familiar with this technology, more cases of suspected AD may come to the attention of medical and social services, and at an earlier stage, with increased requests for new forms of treatment. Patients and care-givers, however, may have their hopes raised from information published on these sites or become distressed when on-line. Intranets may reduce some of these problems, but dealing with the explosion of information may stretch resources to an even greater extent.

Getting information to all groups will require the use of both traditional and new methods of dissemination. Further research to look at effective ways of doing this is still required, given the complexity of the issues. Much can be learnt, though, from current initiatives in Europe; and future prospects for improved access and understanding of information in the new decade are encouraging.

References

1   Dansk Neurologisk Selskab (1997) *Reference Programme for Dementia*. Copenhagen (Danish). In press.

2   Fuhrmann R (1997) *Early Onset Dementia in the Brighton, Hove and Lewes Area: prevalence and service needs*. Brighton Area Branch, Alzheimer Disease Society.

3   Keady J (1996) The experience of dementia: a review of the literature and implications for nursing practice. *J Clin Nursing*. **5**: 275–88.

4   Farmer A (1994) *Littlewick Medical Centre – Caring for carers*. South Derbyshire Health Authority, Derby.

5   Henwood M (1998) *Ignored and invisible? Carers' experience of the NHS*. Carers National Association, London.

6   Pinto JL, Selmes MA and Creado B (1998) *Transnational Analysis of the Socio-economic Impact of Alzheimer's Disease in the European Union: Spanish case*. Universitat Pompeu Fabra, Alzheimer Espana, Fundacio ACE, Barcelona.

7   Bisset AF and MacPherson IA (1996) Patients with dementia: the view from general practice in Grampian. *Health Bulletin*. **54**(1): 32–6.

8 Cavallo M, Coccurullo C, Fattore G and Salvini-Porro G (1998) *Italian country report on Alzheimer's Disease*. Bocconi University and Alzheimer Italia, Milan.

9 Knudsen JL (1998) *Country Report on Alzheimer's Disease in Denmark*. Danish Hospital Institute, Copenhagen.

10 Alzheimer Disease Society (1995) *'Right from the start' Primary Health Care and Dementia: a report by the Alzheimer's Disease Society on the experiences of GPs and carers of dementia diagnoses*. Alzheimer Disease Society, London.

11 Wolff LE, Woods JP and Reid J (1995) Do general practitioners and old age psychiatrists differ in their attitudes to dementia? *Int J Ger Psych*. **10**: 63–9.

12 Lomas J (1993) Diffusion, dissemination and implementation: who should do what? In: KS Warren and F Mosteller (eds) *Doing More Good than Harm: the evaluation of healthcare interventions*. Annals of the New York Academy of Sciences, **703**: 226–41.

13 Fratiglioni L, Nordberg G, Von Strauss E *et al.* (1998) *Swedish Country Report on Alzheimer's Disease*. Institute of Gerontology and the Karolinksa Institute, Stockholm.

14 Von der Schulenberg M and Claes C (1998) *Transnational Analysis of the Socioeconomic Impact of Alzheimer's Disease in the European Union: German report*. University of Hanover.

15 Goes ES, Blom M, Van der Roer N *et al.* (1998) *Dutch Country Report on Alzheimer's Disease*. Erasmus University and the Dutch Alzheimer Society, Rotterdam.

16 Wimo A (1998) Dementia Care: issues for European healthcare systems. *Eurohealth*. **4**(3): 16–17.

17 Scurfield M (1994) What do carers need? *J Dementia Care*. **2**(3): 18–19.

18 Jacques (1994) *Survey of Health Board Provision for Dementia*. Dementia Services Development Centre, University of Stirling.

19 Wright SD, Lund DA, Pett MA and Caserta MS (1987) The assessment of support group experience by caregivers of dementia patients. *Clin Geront*. **6**: 35–9.

20 Dementia Web (2000) http://dementia.ion.ucl.ac.uk/

21 Fearnley K (1997) *Dementia Helpline Annual Report*. Alzheimer Scotland – Action on Dementia, Edinburgh.

22 Dementia Services Development Centre (DSDC) (1999) http://www.stir.ac.uk/Departments/HumanSciences/dsdc/

ERRATUM

Page 175, 1st para, line 2

For 'Coherence' read 'convergence'

9

Towards coherent policy and practice in Alzheimer's disease across the EU

Morton Warner and Sally Furnish

Introduction

The language developed for use within the European Union is constantly evolving. Whilst trying to create economic *harmonisation* and *coherence* undoubtedly has its problems – to introduce two of the buzz-words – they are nothing when compared with those surrounding moves towards political unity and social solidarity, where, until recently, no organising expression existed.

Now it does; and it involves another dynamic piece of code, one which allows for the ebb and flow of ideas and for the *realpolitik*. It is *coherency* – a term not entirely without appeal. But the apparent downside is that, at first glance, it appears as just another Euroword – akin to the Ford Focus with charm, something which means everything and nothing. Therein, of course, lies its attractiveness too, in a developing political scene where clarity is not always helpful!

But this maybe is to belittle an expression which, when examined more closely, proves to be very useful in making a pan-European analysis of the state of play with respect to Alzheimer's disease (AD) policy and practice; and in suggesting how to move ahead, particularly in a Union that is expanding and which will experience even greater cultural diversity.

So, the first part of this chapter will explore the theme of *coherency*, and do so in a way that links it to what Dworkin has referred to as the sovereign virtue, *equality*.[1] What will follow is an analysis of the state of advancement of AD policy and practice in respect of the various subjects covered in earlier chapters: some of the necessarily bald findings will be placed into a broader policy context. The final part will set out ways in which greater coherency could be achieved in a Europe, not just of 15 nations, but which is constantly expanding.

A framework for improvement

The existing membership of the EU is diverse in its political origins, different in terms of cultural perspectives, and varying in levels of development. At the sub-national level the distinctions may be even more stark; and this makes for particular difficulties, because decision making about how policies are to be implemented and programmes of care delivered are very often made here. Indeed, the regional level has been receiving increasing attention from the Commission, and the WHO European Office has formally recognised it in their own restructuring.

Two major reasons exist for the presence of the EU. Put in simple terms, first the members come together out of the economic necessity to create their own trading block as the world quite rapidly develops along these lines. Second, and most important for our purposes here, there is a perception – often under challenge – that Europe should attempt to define for itself what constitutes a civic society in its own terms. Having done so, it should instigate a process of social engineering aimed at overall improvement when set against some grouping of ideals.

For the past 200 years or so the notion of equalitarianism (where a community treats each of its members with equal concern) has featured highly as a rallying cry for the nations which now make up Europe as they formed and reformed, created new alliances, and came to their present relatively stable state. But how is lack of equality to be described?

To paraphrase Dworkin's argument the following formula might be offered:

$$\text{Inequality} \approx \frac{\text{Equal welfare}}{\text{level}} - \frac{\text{Deviation from equal}}{\text{welfare level}} = \text{Equity deficit}$$

A test of whether a policy or programme provides an improvement to the situation comes from a judgement that the equity deficit has been reduced; and this is based on minimising the deviation from the equal welfare level.

The concept of *welfare level* also needs further explanation. It is composed of two parts: in one component it is about resource availability and can, most often, be monetised; and in another it is about liberty. Here, a liberty deficit is related to restrictions of being able to do or to achieve something which in normal circumstances should be possible. This is particularly pertinent to carers of AD sufferers.

The final challenge, then, is to reconcile liberty and equality in order to ensure predominant improvements in the latter. Two possibilities emerge.

A   Reduce equality deficit, related   *but*   do not increase equality
    to resources and liberty of some   deficit of others.

B   No fresh liberty deficits   *but with*   improved resource position
                                                    for group with greatest
                                                    deficit (where any deficit loss
                                                    is less than gain of most
                                                    disadvantaged).

This redistribution approach is at the heart of action stemming from high levels of equality of concern and forms the core of coherence. In formulaic terms it can be displayed as shown in Figure 9.1.

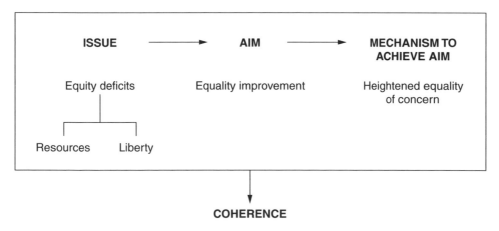

Figure 9.1:   The redistribution approach.

Coherence, then, is different from convergence and is about consistency of approach and reasoning rather than final destinations; and it is more dynamic and flexible in taking into account cultural specificities, and indeed, the way these specificities may change over time.

This formula provides the framework within which to examine AD policy and practice developments across Europe, to venture just a little beyond a crude analysis of rights and wrongs, the comparison of *haves* and *have nots*, and implied criticism of different social systems. It allows appropriate support and encouragement to be constructed by the EU with a lessened sense of victimisation.

Establishing the equal welfare level

The actual situation in which AD sufferers and their carers find themselves in at the beginning of the new century is now examined. First, it is helpful to establish in some way the level that could be set to give a description of 'equal welfare'.

Gathering together the findings across the range of studies represented in this book, certain pan-European principles emerge, which were identified in Chapter 2. These are repeated below (*see* Box 9.1).

Box 9.1:   Key pan-European principles for AD policy

Principles emphasised by *all* member states

1   Sufferers should be able to remain at home for as long as possible
2   Carers should receive as much help as possible, in order to achieve the above
3   Sufferers should retain maximum control over the support they receive
4   *All* relevant services should be co-ordinated at the local level
5   Sufferers in institutional care should live in surroundings which are as 'homely' as possible

---

As such, this list suggests the current *equality of concern*, at least that which exists at the level of ideals, even if not actually representing the practice which many of the contributions suggest.

A second list also has emerged of those items existing on a widespread but not all-encompassing basis (*see* Box 9.2).

Box 9.2:   Key principles for AD care

Principles emphasised by most member states

1   There should be a systematic attempt to equate service provision with need
2   Categorical care should be replaced by care which addresses the general needs of sufferers
3   Early diagnosis of dementia should be encouraged
4   The needs of people with dementia are not addressed separately from the needs of older people in general at the national level

---

Again, the fact that even some states fail to emphasise a principle when most states do indicates some level of equity deficit in Europe. This, added to the policy–practice disjunction, both for this table and the one above, provides a picture of considerable equity deficit.

Deviations from the equal welfare level (the equity deficit)

Resources

At the outset it must be acknowledged that even the identification of older people with dementia is not clear-cut. In some countries, the process by which dementia cases are distinguished from those with physical and mental frailty is uncertain and haphazard. Furnish's conclusion in this respect is to some degree explained later in her analysis of the structural defaults in service provision (*see* Chapter 5). But Lawlor and his colleagues also suggest that an immaturity in clinical training, specialisation and referral mechanisms would contribute (*see* Chapter 6).

The legal status acquired by those with confirmed dementia also has a bearing in some countries, as Gove reminds us (*see* Chapter 3); but without the initial diagnosis, resources cannot be triggered. The balance between the equality of welfare components of resource application and liberty are difficult to resolve.

The more classical equity items which inhibit fairness also come heavily into play – where people live, their age and their socio-economic background. The ETAS study amalgamated the results from six of the European case studies to produce the results shown in Figure 9.2.

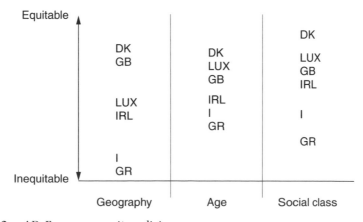

Figure 9.2:   AD: European equity policies.

There is a wide variation of responses.

- In terms of geography, equal access to services varies quite significantly, with the greatest equity deficits in Italy and Greece.
- The ageism spread was not judged to be so wide, but eligibility for services, expressed in implicit and explicit terms, varies, with least certainty for patients and sufferers again in Italy and Greece, but also Ireland.
- Socio-economic discrimination – the failure to provide equality – again shows people in Italy and Greece to be in the worst situation.
- In all three instances Denmark provides the services in a way most close to the equal welfare level, and it also does well in terms of quality of clinical care provision at primary and secondary level.

By way of summary it can be said that dementia care practice is at various stages of development across Europe, with Denmark, Sweden, Finland, the Netherlands and the UK the most mature, but even here joined-up health and social care is not at a high level.

In Portugal, there are no specialised dementia care services, while in Greece there are moves towards setting up some limited services for dementia patients. Other countries, such as Luxembourg and Belgium, have relatively few specific care services dedicated to elderly dementia patients. As a result, patients in those countries are included in the services for the elderly in general. Most countries in Europe are in a transition stage and beginning to develop specialised services. There is still considerable geographical inequity in those countries with services located primarily in urban areas. Only two countries have begun to provide specialised services for patients with pre-senile dementia – the UK and Germany.

In those member states that appear to have more comprehensive dementia services, the issue of variation of service delivery within a country has been recognised as a problem. For example, a change of policy in 1993 in Sweden, allowing municipalities greater discretion in the funding of services for elderly care, has resulted in differences in service provision and eligibility criteria for dementia care between the municipalities. A similar inequity operates in Denmark, but an initiative led by the National Association of Local Authorities is under way to address this problem and to ensure that the same quality in the services can be provided to the different geographical areas. In Ireland, while most health board areas have specialised geriatric services, with assessment and continuing care components for dementia patients, only two health board areas have geriatric psychiatry services.

Liberty

The stages through which AD sufferers go towards their ultimate death causes major differences in this second area of potential equity deficit. Indeed, the major problem identified in policy implementation relates to the uncertainty that prevails. Across Europe, ambiguities and ambivalence exist in abundance, as illustrated in Box 9.3.

Box 9.3: Common criticisms of policy implementation

- Continuing *lack of adequate resources*, particularly resources 'ear-marked' specifically for this client group
- The persistent relatively *low status of dementia services* in the broader context of healthcare
- Inadequate attempts to ensure *patient and carer control* of services, which remain shaped by organisation and professional imperatives
- The health and social needs of *patients and carers* still do not always receive equal attention

---

Liberty for sufferers

Centrally, the liberty deficit was identified earlier as existing when an individual (patient or carer) cannot do or achieve something which in normal circumstances they would find possible. Many of the issues which have crucial liberty elements, and which are brought together below, are dealt with differently across Europe.

- *The right to know* – Here the situation is very mixed indeed. The degree to which doctors reveal an AD diagnosis varies widely; and so does the level of patients wanting to know. Age of the patient is also a factor, with a tendency for older people to have less chance of being informed; and relatives in different countries express varying degrees of agreement to the diagnosis being given to the patient. Some countries have a charter which gives an individual the right to see medical notes on their state of health; and in others the patient is given the right to refuse to receive information about the AD diagnosis. The potential reduction of the liberty deficit is generally low.
- *Guardianship* – Here all EU countries have some kind of law in force. However, the purpose of the arrangement differs. In Spain, there is a reticence to declare incompetence, and formal guardianship levels are

low. In France and the UK, emphasis is on protecting sufferers from
making detrimental decisions. By contrast, Germany and Denmark
require the guardian to help improve the care and personal welfare
of the individual, in positive but rare approaches to reducing the
liberty deficit.

* *Advance directives* – The presence of these provides a freedom of
  decision making about future quality of life and circumstances
  pertaining to death. Not surprisingly, it is three non-Catholic countries – the UK, Holland and Denmark – which have recognised their
  authority, but the ethical debates continue to be lively. The 1997
  European Convention on Human Rights and Biomedicine gives force
  to previously expressed wishes related to medical intervention, but its
  application is patchy in practice and the liberty deficit continues.

* *Everyday living* – Here two items can be scrutinised as indicators:
  employment and driving. Both present difficulties in the areas of
  personal freedom. Clearly, individuals should be able to pursue both
  activities; and the point at which they cannot varies across member states because the onset of AD is unclear, resulting in actions
  not necessarily consistent with the staging of the disease. The liberty deficit varies accordingly. No clear policy picture emerges in
  relation to protection from the consequences of AD or the freedom
  to continue working, and under this situation a liberty deficit is likely
  to exist. The situation is only marginally more clear in respect of
  driving. The UK requires a medical examination and can withdraw the licence, whilst Sweden declines this route. Austria with-
  draws the licence, but reinstates it for local, familiar territory. There
  is little coherence.

It is easy to be critical and to condemn the patchiness of practice across
all these important areas. However, all of them are very complex in
terms of the principles to be debated. But debated they should be, and
on a continuing basis if greater clarity is required. This, in itself, may be
a step too far!

Liberty for carers

A continuing theme throughout earlier chapters has been the important
role played by carers. Indeed, somewhat consistently across Europe, in
spite of different legal obligations, McDaid and Murray have been able
to conclude that the burden of caring (if it is perceived as a burden) is
often accepted, but that support is vital (*see* Chapter 4).

First, then, an overview of these two elements, as shown in Figure 9.3.

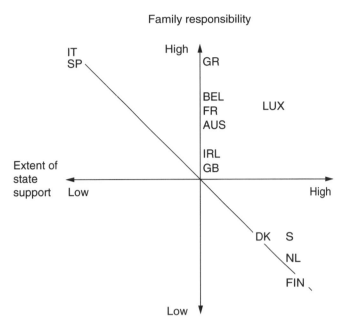

Figure 9.3: Who is responsible for AD care – the state or the family?

The country groupings are quite clear: there is one group, containing the southern members, where state support is low and family responsibility high; another is at the opposite end of the spectrum and is dominated by Scandinavian countries; a third illustrates requirements for a balance between family and state, with the financial onus on the former and care provision on the later. Of the remainder, Ireland and Great Britain follow a muddling through and rather ambivalent approach, while Luxembourg is an outrider, and pursues a rather interesting and balanced pathway.

Each country has responded to its own social and cultural circumstances, set against a backdrop of requirements for economic development. Of course, all of these elements are subject to change and modification.

But the fundamental liberty issue remains. Are carers placed in a position of liberty deficit? In some ways and in some places, the answers are probably 'yes' and 'no'. Luxembourg, alone, seems to have recognised that a balance is necessary between a willingness to accept family responsibility and the need to back this up with state support. However, the Scandinavian groups and the Netherlands have abrogated the family from responsibility which may, in the long term, prove difficult to sustain as pressure is placed upon public financing. The southern group probably over-rely on women to be carers, and this, too, will be increasingly disadvantageous as demography and employment patterns change. These countries, it will be remembered, together with Greece, are also where services are less developed. The remainder appear to be hovering on a policy divide and only time will tell the direction of their future movement.

But to return to the theme of cohesion – there is little, in relation either to resource or liberty equality, and Box 9.4 displays this.

Box 9.4: Policy diversity in continuing care in Europe

Responsibility	Basis of provision	Needs addressed	Eligibility criteria	Form of support

• Individual sufferer
  – personal insurance
  – co-payment
  – full payment
• Family
  – part payment
  – full payment
• Insurance
• Local government
• National government
• Charity/ voluntary organisations
	• Legal requirement
	• Discretionary
		• Specific (e.g. housing)
		• General (e.g. income support)
			• Means tested
			• Universal
				• Cash
				• Services

Every element displays a multiplicity of responses; and these exist for both national and sub-national levels. For carers this must be difficult to understand, and it probably explains the considerable amount of carer literature and NGO developments in the field of AD.

The implications of no action

It is rarely possible in the public policy area to take no action once the ball has been set rolling. The EU, by funding enquiries into this area of AD, has provoked a debate which will not go away; it is now seen to be conjoined with pressure groups across Europe.

But it is not AD *per se* which is at the heart of the debate. Here the emphasis is on the pressure on resources, and demands for better quality of care. Figure 9.4 captures the picture.

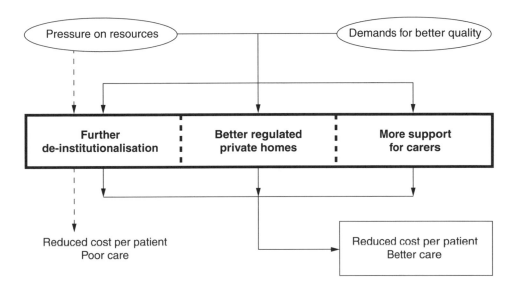

Figure 9.4:   The policy drivers.

Essentially, further de-institutionalisation by itself may lead to reduced costs and certainly will bring poorer care. But the implications of maintaining or improving costs and quality are that action will be required to bring cohesion around the provision of services through care homes and in giving more support to carers.

The way to greater coherency

The purpose of this final section is to highlight the issues which emerge as being of *greatest significance for the EU as a whole*, and to offer concrete proposals to improve the well-being of people with AD and their carers in Europe. Policy-makers and practitioners, both across Europe and in individual member states, will have to judge whether or not AD sufferers and carers have equality of their concern across a number of areas. These are identified below, and coherency recommendations made.

Key issues

AD sufferers and their carers are subject to an equity deficit within member states

The whole context of policy relating to AD is characterised by paradox. On the one hand, there is general recognition that people with the condition (and other dementias) receive a generally poor level of service in comparison with other groups; and yet, on the other hand, there is little sign of impending large-scale improvement. It is upon an understanding of the reasons for this paradox that future progress depends, and part of the answer lies in the low status accorded to this group of people.

Although the member states differ considerably in terms of their policies and services for people with AD and dementia generally, it remains the case that every state accords this client group relatively low status. There are many indicators of this, such as the absence of planning processes and policies specifically targeted at this group, the relatively low prestige enjoyed by many doctors, nurses and other healthcare professionals working with demented patients, and the ambivalent nature – bordering on social stigma – typical of much popular media coverage of dementia, both fact and fiction. This low status underlies many of the other issues identified in succeeding sections.

The causes are many and various. They include:

- the lack of good models of service provision from the past – partly because dementia has only relatively recently become a major public policy issue as the population has aged
- the low prospects of cure for most patients, which tends to conflict with the overriding medical aim (and that of other health professionals) to save life
- the often ambiguous attitude of society at large to its older members – a complex mixture of respect, love and sympathy, coupled with contempt, fear and lack of understanding
- the *invisibility* of the problem, in part a consequence of the marginalised position of most patients, effectively denied a public voice by the consequences of their condition
- the willingness – at least hitherto – of most families of people with dementia to arrange for the care of the affected relative without demanding more resources
- the concern of Ministries of Finance and insurance companies that the burgeoning numbers of demented people, coupled with the low

level of historical provision for them, might lead to an explosion of demand for services which could not easily be afforded.

Many of the above are, of course, interrelated, but together they form the elements to which greater attention is needed.

The proportion of professional staff specialising in dementia shows a high degree of national variation, which appears to be related to the level of economic development of the country. In all countries, however, most of the staff caring for people with AD and related disorders, whether in domiciliary or residential/nursing settings, are untrained and poorly supervised. They are generally regarded as of low status, despite the numerous challenges of their work, and recruitment is difficult. Most of the workforce comprises unqualified nurses, care workers or members of charitable and religious organisations. Staffing ratios are often unfavourable, yet there is known to be a considerable degree of *burn-out* in working with people with high levels of mental and physical dependency.

Identifying a community of interest in relation to people with AD and related disorders from a national perspective has proved to be a challenge in itself. The AD societies came closest to playing this role. If one compares this situation with the community of interest around people with learning disabilities, for example, where in many countries a number of stakeholders have developed a common set of demands, dementia is still a long way behind. A community of interest encourages an ongoing examination of how values related to the group in question are upheld in services. The formation of a community of interest generally occurs when groups of people with disabilities are more formally acknowledged. The reported lack of specific AD policies, together with general concerns that the growing numbers of sufferers will be overwhelming, may well be related to this finding.

- *Coherency 1* – There should be a concerted attempt, both at national and European levels, to use the most effective means of public education to change negative attitudes towards AD, and in particular to emphasise the benefits to be derived from early diagnosis.
- *Coherency 2* – Member states should use whatever policy levers they have available to them to increase the professional status of healthcare staff working with demented patients, and professional bodies themselves should develop strategies to achieve the same ends.
- *Coherency 3* – As part of the strategy to raise the status of AD services, member states should encourage the development of local, regional and national 'communities of interest' for AD which bring together all the relevant stakeholders. The Commission should consider providing a degree of European co-ordination to such efforts.

There is equity deficit between member states in dealing with AD

It is often difficult to compare the quality of healthcare provision across Europe, given the very different organisational and philosophical contexts in which the member states work. In the case of AD, however, such comparisons are made somewhat easier by the fact that there is such a high degree of agreement on the basic characteristics of good policy and service provision. It is possible, therefore, to map the extent to which individual states fall short of the ideal.

There are many examples of inequity of provision of dementia care across the EU. Clinical practice models are quite advanced in some countries but are embryonic and at an early stage of development in others. Even where dementia care practice is well developed, there is often geographical inequity in the provision of such services, or imbalances in the level of specialist provision that translate into inequity for the sufferers and their carers. In most member states, primary care personnel are significantly under-trained and under-resourced to deal with the rising tide of dementia sufferers, contributing to the late detection and treatment of these disorders.

Funding mechanisms, drug reimbursement procedures and prescribing for new drug treatments in AD vary from country to country and represent another source of inequity for patients and their carers. AD and dementia are unique among the leading causes of chronic disability and ill health in that the sufferers themselves are often not able to act as advocates for the treatment of their condition. This may partly account for the low priority given in some member states to the funding of new treatments and interventions for this condition.

The degree of standardisation of service responses to AD also varies between countries. For example, the same clinical presentation may lead to a referral to support services in one region but not in another part of the same country. The reasons for this seem to be less to do with the financial systems involved in paying for health and social care and more related to the process of interpretation of national policy into priorities to be actioned at local level.

For those countries where needs had been estimated, the task was not made easier by the absence of a consensus around definitions of AD and related disorders. International and national studies provide estimates of prevalence, although it is rarely possible to estimate incidence. There is widespread concern about the process of interpreting when a dementing illness constitutes a need, especially a health need. Countries with policies of universal access to healthcare are especially concerned about how to meet increasing demand as a result of demographic changes and the licensing of new medications.

No state has a perfect level of provision, and there is room for improvement in all. It is also true, however, that some have managed to develop better provision than others. This is often explained by such basic issues as the strength of the local economy (as a key determinant of the level of expenditure on welfare). But whatever the cause, there is a clear *prima facie* need for co-ordination of services and policies to reduce current inequities.

*   *Coherency 4* – The Commission should work with member states to provide assistance to those whose services for AD are furthest from the ideal level of provision.
*   *Coherency 5* – Member states should review (and where necessary improve) the consistency of local application of nationally-accepted and community-wide good practice in relation to AD.

Intervention often occurs at too late a stage in the progress of AD

The intellectual and humanitarian case for early identification of people with AD is by now well-established. And yet many policy-making organisations, as well as individual practitioners, still do not accept the case; or if they do, they seem unable or unwilling to bring it about. This is partly a consequence of the generally low status of AD. But there are also more specific causes. Many professionals lack the relevant skills or time to perform the differential diagnosis necessary, or can see little point in so doing, given their orientation towards saving lives. There may also be argument that the patient's best interests – in terms of preserving their dignity or confidentiality – are not served by making an early diagnosis. Relatives, too, will often collude with professionals and request that the diagnosis not be disclosed to the patient, further underscoring family members' negative attitudes to AD.

*   *Coherency 6* – The relevant agencies in each member state should develop an effective strategy to increase the level and quality of assessment and diagnosis of AD at the early stages of the disease, and should consider setting targets to this end.
*   *Coherency 7* – Each member state should also ensure that general medical and allied professional education includes sufficient input on dementia at undergraduate, postgraduate and continuing education levels.

AD policy should be co-ordinated, and the services provided should be multidisciplinary

Service provision provides the ultimate test of policy integrity. A lack of specific recognition of AD and related disorders has been reported across the EU, despite considerable growth in the carers' movement generally and the fact that the social consequences of cognitive impairment have been highlighted.

AD patients have a multiplicity of different, and often quite intractable, problems. There is much attention paid now to the need for multi-disciplinary health and social care, and for the application of both medical and social models of care – and nowhere is this more needed than in the case of services for people with AD. A whole range of professional disciplines must be brought to bear at the appropriate junctures, including (where they exist) general practitioners, community psychiatric nurses, domiciliary nurses, health visitors/public health nurses, social workers, old age psychiatry services, geriatricians, psychiatrists, neurologists and other therapists. It is not that multi-agency dementia services do not exist, but that policies frequently do not support their development or continuation, and other priority groups take precedence. The literature is abundant with good demonstration projects for dementia services in a number of countries, but the indications are that they have not had a pronounced impact on policy.

Particular problems have been revealed in generating preventive approaches for the *social* consequences of cognitive impairment in elderly people – a failure to take account of the uniqueness of a dementing illness like AD. Multi-agency working can greatly improve the prospect of the totality of the patient's needs being properly addressed.

The best match of service to need will often be achieved by addressing the issue of appropriate specialisation. All European healthcare systems depend to some extent upon generalist professionals identifying the healthcare needs of the population, and meeting most of those needs themselves. In the case of AD, generalists must be able and willing to perform the majority of assessments, and to provide continuity of care to the patient and their carers through the progression of their disease. If they are to fulfil this role effectively, however, they must also have easy access to the sorts of specialist services which it would not be practicable to provide at the primary care level. Deficiencies in both sectors must be addressed simultaneously. Policies directed towards co-ordinating services through a form of primary care, together with social care planning and defined pathways into secondary specialist services, are particularly important components in the development of the future direction of services.

At present it is relatively uncommon for institutional services to deliver individualised care irrespective of the level of severity of the person's problems. If most staff providing direct care are untrained in the effects of dementia, there is a tendency to believe, in line with popular misconception, that the difficult behaviour often displayed by people with dementia is deliberate. Such beliefs are associated with dehumanising care practices. In member states where the balance is still towards large-scale institutional care, there is a case for making institutional care the last resort when all other attempts to support the person through formal services in their own home have failed.

Policy-makers, too, need to work across boundaries for this particular group of people. In fact, many government departments formulate and implement policy which can improve – or make more difficult – the lives of people with AD and their carers. Such departments include social security, transport, and housing, as well as the more obvious health and social services sectors. Most member states have examples of where policy formulated for another group – such as those with physical disabilities – is being applied in an *ad hoc* way to the circumstances of those with dementia, with the inevitable results. What is needed is policy specifically formulated to meet the unique circumstances of dementia, and which embraces all relevant departments and agencies.

Again, one returns to the issue of priorities: co-ordination could be achieved, if only it were accorded sufficient priority amongst policy-makers and service providers. The pre-existing boundaries, which make little sense from the perspective of AD patients and their carers, usually serve other – valid – administrative purposes. Therefore the objective should be either to develop mechanisms for bridging the divides in this instance, or to create entirely new arrangements for patients with dementia. The preferred option will depend upon the individual local circumstances, but the degree of priority should universally be high.

It would also help national governments if there were more effective means of disseminating throughout Europe the lessons of practice development and models of organisation in individual countries.

- *Coherency 8* – Member states should continue to address the need to improve co-ordination – at the policy and implementation levels – to meet the total needs of AD patients and their carers.
- *Coherency 9* – The balance between generalist and specialist provision should be revised in each member state, in order to ensure that both are fulfilling their most appropriate roles.
- *Coherency 10* – A mechanism should be established to evaluate and disseminate across Europe new models of service delivery and organisation.

Carers of AD sufferers require better support

The support available to family care-givers is widely reported to be inadequate, despite the evidence of effectiveness of some psycho-educational approaches with informal carers. In the more economically deprived countries, families perform the majority of care in the absence of alternatives, and without explicit consideration of the emotional costs to both sufferer and carer of the consequences of such a policy. In other member states, family carers have the right to apply for support or to request an assessment of their needs. The disincentives to applying for support of a financial, practical or emotional nature are reported to be high in most countries which make provision for informal carers. The impression is also given that despite the Alzheimer's disease societies actively performing the role of carers' pressure groups, little carer participation in service planning takes place.

Research evidence indicates that the carers of elderly people with dementia have poorer physical and emotional health than carers of elderly people who are equally dependent but less affected by deteriorating mental capacity. Also, a higher proportion of family-caring situations break down irretrievably when the carer of an elderly person with dementia becomes unwell themselves for a period of time. Frequently the crisis response of services is less effective in maintaining the person with dementia than is the family care-giver, and this is even true of elderly spouse carers. It is very much in the best interests of services to support any existing carers before they cease to be able to cope.

- *Coherency 11* – There should be further improvements in the systematic identification of the needs of carers, supported by the allocation of adequate resources to meet their (often modest) requirements.
- *Coherency 12* – All member states should continue to improve the mechanisms used to involve carers.

If a co-ordinated and sustained approach is developed, which addresses the coherency agenda set out above, the prospects for a more humane society in Europe will become a reality. Few families and individuals will not benefit from the health protection that will be provided.

Reference

1   Dworkin R (2000) *Sovereign Virtue: the theory and practice of equality.* Harvard University Press, Cambridge.

Index